The Concise Guide
to Decision Making
and Ethics
in Dysphagia

British Library Cataloguing in Publication Data

A catalogue record for this book is available from the British Library

Cover design: Jim Wilkie

Cover image: by 'clivewa' used under license from Shutterstock.com

Project management, typesetting and design: J&R Publishing Services Ltd, Guildford, Surrey, UK; www.jr-publishingservices.co.uk

The Concise Guide to Decision Making and Ethics in Dysphagia

Paula Leslie and Hannah Crawford

J&R Press Ltd

Contents

Foreword

Dysphagia, or the study of abnormal swallowing, is struggling toward maturity. Case studies, personal accounts of difficulty and frustration, small group studies of groups – stroke patients, those with Parkinson's disease, and others – descriptions of treatments supported by clinical intuition, patient report and a modicum of data – often from normal swallowers – and first-person accounts of how-to-do evaluation, often supported by a prescription for selected procedures of unknown validity and reliability, dominated the literature and guided both researchers and clinicians during the field's infancy. Small – but larger than in the beginning – group studies of more carefully and homogenously selected groups of both normal and abnormal swallowers, psychometric data on a host of approaches to evaluation, treatment development from confirmation of biological action to randomized clinical trials, linkage of pathophysiology and treatment approach, attempted replications of treatment studies, and identification of dysphagia in an array of both common and uncommon conditions confirmed the field's systematic growth. Unfortunately, outbursts of immaturity such as indiscriminate use of untested treatments continue to occur but with decreased frequency and wider and more immediate public censure. Books, biographies of the profession's growth, jostle for a place on the devices or shelves of researchers and clinicians alike. Professional calendars bulge with workshops, and special, interdisciplinary societies provide a sense of shared purpose. Professionals can be forgiven for thinking their profession is now mature and that traditional, comfortable activities, refined by additional data and experience, will prevent premature decline.

The Concise Guide to Decision Making and Ethics in Dysphagia by Leslie, a PhD with a Master's in bioethics and a history of clinical practice, and Crawford, a PhD who describes herself as a clinician "through and through," outlines a different future, one requiring putting the patient and ethical decision making on the same level as the patient's swallow, the clinician's viewpoint, and physiologically-based evaluation and treatment planning. The authors portray the complexity of eating, drinking and swallowing disorders and focus on how the clinician and patient/family might work together more effectively to make decisions: balancing clinical evidence, patient preferences and ethical principles. This role of ethical principles in decision making is only recently, tentatively and incompletely being incorporated into clinical practice by health care professionals, including speech-language pathologists. This book will hasten and strengthen that incorporation.

I can imagine howls of protest from those whose careers have been spent measuring normal and abnormal swallows in a variety of populations and under a variety of conditions, who nod knowingly when clinicians are described as mechanical engineers, who applaud the descriptions and promise of more sophisticated transducers and non-invasive measures of nervous system function, who argue that a treatment's value rests with its biological activity-skill building, strengthening-and who consider a treatment's (and clinician's) legitimacy as resting solely on successfully matching underlying pathophysiology and each method's active ingredients. Moreover, continues the protest I am imagining, practice is – and forever has been – guided by ethical principles long established by professional associations such as the American Speech Language and Hearing Association. Thus ethical principles – a positive treatment outcome cannot be guaranteed for example – are inherent in modern practice and if they are not then professional punishment is swift.

Ethics, and specifically bioethics as discussed in their book, are both more than and in most ways different from what the majority of practitioners appear to be talking about on the few occasions they mention ethics as part of management at all. For Paula and Hannah, bioethics is an "area of ethical study concerned with issues in healthcare, life sciences and clinical research" (p.23), and "The role of bioethics may be thought of as using ethical concepts to help clinicians, and more broadly policymakers and researchers, make decisions." Sounds pretty easy and non-threatening on the surface. Permission to treat documents and explaining the treatment methodology and expected outcomes satisfy the principle of autonomy, physiologically oriented treatments guided by data and refined in the crucible of experience guarantee beneficence and nonmaleficence. Justice, or supplying "what people *need* in a *fair* way," seems easy as well. Physiologically-based treatments at the appropriate intensity and duration often improve swallowing safety and allow advances in diet as judged by the clinician. And therein lies one of the problems of present dysphagia management according to the authors – restrictive clinician control over evaluation, treatment and outcome measurement. The authors say it best: "We would argue that we cannot hope to offer person-centred, appropriate assessments or interventions without considering our patients' difficulties in their broader world perspective" (p.19). In their view all clinical decisions rest on two pillars, physiology and bioethics, and when the two fail to support a common decision, the ethical takes precedence. In other words, a sound physiologic decision is not necessarily an ethical decision.

Leslie and Crawford have rich clinical experiences and clinical souls. They know that adding another layer of complexity to an already complex practice wherein even the most experienced of us is never sanguine that any decision is right will be met by resistance or at least scepticism. Thus in seven chapters they provide guidelines for ethical practice and they fold vignettes into the text to demonstrate ethical decision making. Nor are they scolds. I am a better clinician for having read the book, not because they told me I must do better but because they make doing better attractive.

John C. Rosenbek, PhD
Professor Emeritus
University of Florida
Adjunct Professor
Michigan State University

1 Setting the scene

Introduction

We know what causes swallow problems, and what we might do biomechanically and physiologically to address the issues. We can recite the mantra of evidence-based practice: best available evidence, patient beliefs and values, informed clinical expertise. And yet still the world of dysphagia care is populated by clinicians having sleepless nights wondering "was that the right clinical decision, could we have done something else, was this right for the patient and their loved ones, have I discharged my duty of care" and, sadly, "have I done my job properly – could I get sued for malpractice?"

This book outlines why decisions are difficult, what frameworks might help structure more robust decisions, and links evidence to ethics to cases. How can we use theoretical principles of risk analysis and bioethics to support clinical care and the clinicians dealing with patients and their families and carers on a day-to-day basis?

As medical science progresses more people are living longer with more complex medical needs. There has been a corresponding rise in the prevalence of swallowing disorders which clearly cut to the core of health (nutrition and hydration) and, equally importantly, the psychosocial importance of mealtimes and their communality. We know a lot about what causes swallow problems, what we might do to fix or ameliorate things from a biomechanical or physiological perspective. So why are decisions and intervention still fraught with tension, anxiety and sometimes even conflict? The interplay between clinician, patient and caregivers has not progressed to a place where decisions come easy.

There are few texts that address the complexity of decision making as the focus in dysphagia rather than the biomechanics, the assessment or the treatment. Texts almost always come from the clinical scientific perspective of the 'swallow expert'. We will not address physiology, medical signs and symptoms and their meaning, complex comorbidity or pharmacology; there are many good papers and texts on these issues and such topics are invariably clinician-centric.

This text outlines the complexity of eating, drinking and swallowing disorders, and focuses on how the clinician and patient/family might work more effectively together to make decisions: balancing clinical evidence, patient preferences and ethical principles. It is only recently that this last component of formal ethical considerations is being reflected upon and incorporated into clinical reality by healthcare professionals.

How does swallowing become a medical issue?

Swallowing is a fundamental biological process. At its most focused it is the action by which we close off the breathing channel and open the food channel, both of whose entrances are in the same 15cm tube: the pharynx. In under one second, the structures in this space need to be radically altered in position to ensure the cessation of breathing and the initiation and completion of moving a bolus of food or water past the entrance to the airway (the larynx) and into the oesophagus.

This rapid, risky process takes place in a larger framework of feeding, which is part of the psychosocial activity of eating and drinking. We start to think about swallowing possibly as soon as we contemplate an activity involving food or drink such as the first cup of tea or coffee of the day, a cold beer at a barbeque, slicing and eating a piece of wedding cake (Leopold & Kagel, 1997). Cortical involvement relative to food and drink can be mediated even by someone saying "cheddar cheese" or "body odour" (de Araujo, Rolls, Velazco, Margot, & Cayeux, 2005) so it is not much of a stretch to connect thoughts of eating and drinking with how the body might prepare for and execute swallowing.

Swallowing can only start if we can get the food or drink to our mouths. One might argue that being able to manoeuvre food and drink before it touches the lips is an inherent part of the swallow process. Studies of patients based in hospitals and residential settings have shown that simple issues like fatigue affect more people than an impairment in the swallow itself and having a diagnosis might help matters simply because people will pay more attention to you (Westergren, Ohlsson, & Hallberg, 2002).

Once the food and drink has reached the mouth we must then control and manipulate the liquid or solid material into a cohesive bolus that can be passed from the mouth, through the pharynx and into the oesophagus. For this we need teeth - or some way of tearing and softening the food - and the tongue to manoeuvre the emerging bolus around the mouth and back into the pharynx. The volitional swallow moves to a non-volitional process which may also be impaired. This non-volitional process continues down the oesophagus, into the stomach and on through the intestines, and finally as waste product output. We mention this because, although the world of the swallow expert focuses on the oropharyngeal structures and processes, we need to understand that impairments further down the line can affect our patients' eating and drinking.

In this text we are deliberately vague in our case vignettes. We do not give detail about the type of stroke that our patient has, or what medications they are on. These details should be addressed by the competent clinician in the disease evaluation and treatment planning. The myriad of specifics would lead this text into the realm of the traditional text: anatomy- and physiology-centric. We wish to focus our readers' attention on process, on global factors, and to encourage self-reflection at a metacognitive level. What do I know and what do I not know about my patient that I should know? What information is missing? How do the mechanics of the physiological problem translate for this patient with their social unit, with their wants and goals, with the resources of both the clinical service and the patient?

The focus of our attention

At the centre of our focus is the individual with a swallowing problem, be they a patient, client or service user. The term used is dependent upon current fashion, political correctness and clinical care setting. There is much debate not only about the negativity of the medical model and the word 'patient' but also the commercialization of health and aligning our populations with business 'clients' or 'service users'. We will use the term 'patient' in this text given that speech and language therapy (and other professionals involved in swallowing disorders) is a clinical profession. 'Patient' also allows us to avoid the confusion over who exactly the 'client' is in a decision making process as it will refer to the individual with dysphagia.

In school, we focus very much on the patient being the centre of our world. Then as we practise in the real world we gain an appreciation of the family and their role. We need to continue this development by understanding that families (and friends and healthcare professionals) can help the patient to make decisions and that any decisions made by the patient also affect the families.

In most cases there will be significant others who may be family members or those who have a bond of friendship over the years, or even health and social care workers. Biological or legal family members will be called 'family carers' to distinguish them from those carers (who will be termed 'professional carers') who have developed a relationship (which might be very strong) as a result of their professional position. Friends should also be remembered as possible major contributors to a person's wellbeing. Friends may bring a long history of knowledge and intimate discussions which some people would never have with family.

What decisions need to be made?

Some of the difficult decisions our patients and their loved ones may need to consider include:

- To eat or not to eat (the Nil By Mouth debate)
- To place a feeding tube or not to place a feeding tube
- To use thickeners in drinks
- To modify foods
- To change environment to make mealtimes more conducive
- To accept support at mealtimes
- To use adapted cutlery.

Some of these may seem to be small changes. When individuals become dysphagic, eating and drinking becomes a clinical, biomechanical problem. This overrides our ability to engage in relationships, religious and symbolic rites and celebrations. The challenge is that, as clinicians, we are not trained to take this into account. We continue to puzzle over why cases are not as they are presented in the dysphagia textbooks we read during our education. This may be due to the historical and current focus on the biomechanics.

We need to ensure that we carry out our duty of care as health practitioners, but we need to ensure we get it right for each individual patient, their family, friends and care staff. This requires us to view patients equally as socially connected humans and not just bodies that need fuel. Our work must also be framed in the contemporary clinical situation of ever-shrinking resources – both human and financial. Continuing the shift to a more collaborative approach aligns us with best practice and increasingly patient-centric decision making. Increasing patients' activation in their own care (or that of family members) improves health outcomes and the healthcare experience, and is related to lower costs (Hibbard & Greene, 2013; Hibbard, Greene, & Overton, 2013).

The nature of certainty and prognosis

Prognostication is the hardest thing in medicine even after thousands of years. We can create intelligent artificial limbs controlled by brain implants, we can image down to cell level, bring people back from heart and respiratory failure, but we cannot predict with certainty most clinical outcomes. Thus the clinical world can rarely answer the patient's question of "how long do I have, doctor?" or "which treatment is best?" We have growing evidence that families' alleged misinterpretation of clinical advice in the face of the odds/ probability statements that the clinical world offers is less that the family misunderstands and more that they have a drive to remain optimistic (Zier, Sottile, Hong, Weissfield, & White, 2012).

When we combine our lack of prognostic certainty with the human drive of optimism, decision making becomes much more complex. Patients may wish to fight more for their loved ones than for themselves and so suffer inner conflict in the face of these uncertainties. And when asked to decide on behalf of another person, families need to remain optimistic in the face of great odds because they do not want to give up – to lose their loved one. Healthcare professionals may view patients' families as having unrealistic expectations or even meddling in treatment. This is a poor dynamic for all parties involved in decision making.

Limitations

We acknowledge that across the world there are major cultural and legal differences as to how healthcare is viewed and provided; for example, is it a right or a benefit for purchase, who should pay, who should treat, and what should be treated. Scopes of Practice vary across the world even within the one profession, be that speech and language therapy (speech-language pathology), occupational therapy, or ear, nose and throat physicians. What we have set out to do is raise issues for consideration, provide frameworks and resources, and ask questions that address the issues underlying ethical decision making in dysphagia. Ethical decisions are bounded by the context in which they arise. Thus our intent is to enable clinicians to identify issues, options and inappropriacies where perhaps before they would not have been able to do. This transcends local policy and institutional structure whilst acknowledging that they must be addressed.

Case vignettes

We outline here our 'family' of cases that we will return to throughout the book.

Case 1 Henry

Henry is 24 years old with profound and multiple learning and physical difficulties as a result of quadriplegic cerebral palsy. Henry uses a wheelchair and needs help from other people for all aspects of his care and activities of daily living. It is difficult to determine how much Henry can see and hear but he does turn towards loud noises, he sometimes tracks familiar people as they walk across the room, and he sometimes smiles when familiar people come close to him. Henry does not use verbal communication but can vocalize. Familiar staff and family can identify some of his moods from his vocalizations. Henry lives at home with his parents who are in their early 60s. His mother has never worked, and his father recently retired.

Henry attends a social care day centre Monday–Friday, as he has done since he left school four years ago. He receives regular respite care from a non-nursing residential care provider. Henry has a very low weight (approximately 35kgs/77lbs). Henry has recently begun coughing regularly on food and drink. While his parents say that he does not suffer from respiratory infections, the staff who know him well at the day centre say that his chest sounds rattly, that he often looks grey in pallor and is very tired, and there are concerns that his parents do not take him to the doctor to be checked out. The care staff report that his meals take a long time, sometimes over an hour, and that he coughs on all food and drink. When he is eating or drinking they say that a lot of food and drink falls out of his mouth. Henry's parents report no concerns with his eating and drinking. They say that Henry has always been the same and that you just have to know how to feed him. They report that they have not taken Henry to the doctor for at least two years which they feel is a good thing and a sign of his good health.

Case 2 Geethu-Joseph

Geethu-Joseph is from Kerala in southern India. She is in her 70s, widowed and a practising Catholic. Geethu-Joseph has very little spoken English so communication is done via the family. Up until her recent stroke she was an active member of the family unit, particularly with regard to food preparation. Now Geethu-Joseph is cared for by her youngest son's wife. Culture and religion add much to the complexity of this case. Geethu-Joseph had full capacity before her stroke and she said to family (but never wrote down) that she wanted 'everything done'. After the stroke, Geethu-Joseph's communication and cognitive abilities are severely impaired and she cannot make her needs known.

Case 3 Nan

Nan is 75 years old and has Alzheimer's type dementia. She lives in a specialized dementia care facility on the outskirts of an industrial town. Nan's husband has visited her every day since she moved into the facility. This move was very difficult for him as they have been married for 55 years. They had a very close and happy relationship. They had two children who died in an accident when they were teenagers. Nan has a sister and a brother, both of whom work full time, and have their own families. Her brother lives a long way away and visits infrequently. Her sister lives 50 miles away and visits about once a month. Nan speaks fondly of her brother and her sister.

Until recently Nan lived a full and busy life. She attended a ladies group once a week where she and her friends undertook craft projects for charity.

She was also part of a drama group that staged performances for the local community twice a year. Nan loves Elvis Presley and enjoys following a local entertainer who does an Elvis tribute act. Nan once visited Graceland with her husband and enjoys reminiscing about this trip regularly. Nan usually enjoys helping with the housework in the care facility when people will let her – some staff are more understanding of this than others. She particularly likes to help the staff plan and shop for meals, and her designated job is to make the beds in the house. Recently, Nan has become more forgetful, and less motivated to attend her activities and groups.

Case 4 David

David is 48 years old with a wife (Abigail) and two teenage children and until very recently he was a practising engineer. David and his wife are Jewish, they attend services and celebrate the major holidays. They keep Kosher and are keen amateur cooks and have an allotment (community garden). David has cancer – he has had aggressive treatment which slowed the disease for a while but there is no curative intervention. David has weeks/months to live without further aggressive treatment and he has decided that he does not want any more surgery, radio or chemotherapy. David's pain is fairly well controlled. Although he thinks of himself as modern, he has been reflecting on his life and why things happen since the cancer was deemed terminal. He thinks a lot about how to handle pain. David is having increasing difficulty with swallowing and the clinical team has proposed that he considers a gastric feeding tube. Abigail is very supportive of this idea. David is keeping silent on the decision at present.

Case vignette summary

Chapter	Henry PMLD No capacity	Geethu-Joseph CVA No/limited capacity	Nan Dementia Limited capacity	David Cancer Full capacity
1 Introduction				
2 Food culture		X		X
3 Bioethics			X	X
4 Families	X			X
5 Formal care	X		X	
6 Frameworks	X	X		

References

de Araujo, I.E., Rolls, E.T., Velazco, M.I., Margot, C., & Cayeux, I. (2005). Cognitive modulation of olfactory processing. *Neuron*, 46(4), 671-679. doi: 10.1016/j.neuron.2005.04.021

Hibbard, J.H. & Greene, J. (2013). What the evidence shows about patient activation: Better health outcomes and care experiences; fewer data on costs. *Health Affairs*, 32(2), 207-214. doi: 10.1377/hlthaff.2012.1061

Hibbard, J.H., Greene, J., & Overton, V. (2013). Patients with lower activation associated with higher costs: Delivery systems should know their patients' 'scores'. *Health Aff* (Millwood), 32(2), 216-222. doi: 10.1377/hlthaff.2012.1064

Leopold, N.A. & Kagel, M.C. (1997). Dysphagia - ingestion or deglutition?: A proposed paradigm. *Dysphagia*, 12(4), 202-206.

Westergren, A., Ohlsson, O., & Hallberg, I.R. (2002). Eating difficulties in relation to gender, length of stay, and discharge to institutional care, among patients in stroke rehabilitation. *Disability & Rehabilitation*, 24(10), 523-533.

Zier, L.S., Sottile, P.D., Hong, S.Y., Weissfield, L.A., & White, D.B. (2012). Surrogate decision makers' interpretation of prognostic information: A mixed-methods study. *Annals of Internal Medicine*, 156(5), 360-366. doi: 10.7326/0003-4819-156-5-201203060-00008

2 Food, culture, symbolism

Food and mealtimes are important, culturally and symbolically, across all peoples and societies. The variety of meanings associated with food and mealtimes is diverse. Food and drink are essential for survival, for nutrition and hydration. This is the biological process referred to in Chapter 1. Food, drink and mealtimes also play other equally important non-biological roles. These include roles associated with aspects of identity such as family, class, religion and gender. The eating of food and mealtimes are important settings for the socialization of children because they happen regularly and are bound by rules and rituals.

Food and mealtimes also have important cultural and religious functions. You only need to ask a friend "what did you do at Christmas/Diwali/Eid al-Fitr/Rosh Hashanah?" and it is likely that you will be regaled with a story about what time people get up, who is there, what they wear, what ceremony they may take part in and where, whether people exchange gifts. Most important is often what is eaten or drunk, how and when, who prepares the food, maybe what utensils are used to serve and eat with, as this is often the focus of the day. The establishment of national identity is also tied up with food as can be seen in countries that have seen recent political and social change such as Belize. Dishes that had been brought to the country by other cultures were suddenly proclaimed as *Belizean* and great attention was paid to foods that might have been consumed by the indigenous population (Wilk, 1999).

In this chapter we consider some of the main areas in society and for individuals where food plays a major part. These are especially important to consider when an individual has difficulties with eating and drinking.

Identity

There are many different aspects that comprise an individual's identity. In most western societies it is claimed that it is important and desirable to eat as a family (Cason, 2006; Neumark-Sztainer, Hannan, Story, Croll, & Perry, 2003; Neumark-Sztainer, Story, Ackard, Moe, & Perry, 2000; Ochs & Shohet, 2006), although the definition of a 'traditional' family mealtime is not clear (Fiese, Foley, & Spagnola, 2006). Mealtimes tend to be times where families come together and display and reinforce their group membership. The importance of food has been described as: "to both solidify group membership and to set groups apart" (Mintz & Du Bois, 2002, p. 109). There are rules and rituals that are played out within families which may include who is present and where they sit, what utensils are used, what is eaten, who has cooked the food and what is discussed. Families may talk about other people they know, there may be family jokes and traditions. Mealtimes are not always convivial occasions and much stress can be experienced by those responsible for cooking, interfamily tensions and guilt at which sector of the extended family to visit. Mealtime settings have their individual rules, rituals and routines which mark out membership of the group. Mealtimes also serve to build relationships and structures in non-traditional families such as gay, lesbian and transgender units (Carrington, 1999).

The personal aspects of an individual's identity are often associated with food: whether they like to cook, are they a good cook, what they like to eat, what they like to drink, preferences for healthy/exotic food, whether they enjoy eating with friends and family, and whether celebrating is associated with eating food. We all have a relationship with food and an identity that is linked and in some way defined by food.

Gender roles

One of the key aspects of identity is associated with gender, and in particular with respect to the roles involved in the provision of food. We need to reflect on gender roles in the context of the person eating and the person providing food for others. Male family members play important and changing roles with regards to food and mealtimes (Meah, 2014) but the majority of studies look at the role of women in association with food, mealtimes and the preparation and provision of food. Gender and power roles are often displayed and reinforced through the medium of mealtimes (Grieshaber, 1997). Some authors associate the preparation and provision of food with the female sex because of the ability women have to produce milk and feed their children in the act of breastfeeding (Warin, Turner, Moore, & Davies, 2008). While men undoubtedly play a part in mealtimes, lots of the tasks in *feeding work* including planning, preparing, delivering, eating and clearing remain primarily associated with women (Hocking, Wright-St. Clair, & Bunrayong, 2002; Pan, Hsieh, & Wahlqvist, 2009; Warde & Hetherington, 1994).

Feeding work is not always described or experienced as being one of oppression. Women report taking pleasure in providing their family with food, and see the meal as a gift to their loved ones (Fjellström, 2008; Hocking et al., 2002).

This resonates with our clinical experience where mothers report that they prefer to 'hold on' to feeding their adult children with disabilities, as it is such an intimate activity. Mothers also report that they do not trust others to prepare or provide the right type of food for their children. For some groups and individuals, the responsibilities associated with *food work* give women 'culinary capital' and power and we need to consider the context when reflecting on gender roles for women (D'Sylva & Beagan, 2011; Meah, 2014).

Gender roles should not be presumed with any family. Increasingly, families do not follow the male:female two parent nuclear model. Many families have one parent performing multiple roles, or extended structures with relatives or other close adults acting as parents. Lesbian, gay and transgender families use food work and meals as a way of identifying family roles (Carrington, 1999).

In many families there is usually one person who takes on the role of meal planner, figuring out what others like, or need. This is part of the *emotion work* associated with food and it may be undertaken by anyone. It is important to bear in mind that such work goes on behind the scenes for every individual that we come into contact with as practitioners, and our intervention has consequences for these people as well as the patient.

Feeding others

As life begins, feeding is usually associated with the relationship between mother and child. Nursing an infant has been described as "our first and most intimate feeding experience" (Miller, Rozin, & Fiske, 1998, p. 424). In the first few months of an infant's life a primary and important focus is feeding and this period is also a time of intimate communication between the feeder and the infant. This focus on food and feeding continues throughout the child's life (Pan et al., 2009).

During the early years a child requires complete feeding, a task which is considered important and consuming in terms of time and energy. Following the development of competence in eating and being fed, the natural progression is for the carer to help the child learn to feed him or herself which is an important milestone in the child's life. The importance of the feeder role for the carer is retained, but rather than directly feeding the child the emphasis often shifts to providing the right sort of food. In the western world, the issue of "serving healthy food is a strong part of cultural conventions of feeding" (Anving & Thorsted, 2010, p. 30). Feeding the child the right sort of food is associated with the construct of a *good mother* (Bugge & Almås, 2006; Charles & Kerr, 1988; DeVault, 1991; Moisio, Arnould, & Price, 2004).

Moving away from the feeding relationship between parent and child, we need to think about the issue of adult feeding adult, as this is pertinent to our consideration of dysphagia. In adulthood, feeding others is considered to be an intimate act between people. Women have been reported to be more comfortable with the intimacy required for feeding than men (Miller et al., 1998). Miller suggests that this may be due to women commonly undertaking the task of feeding children and that, as a result, feeding may have meaning associated with caretaking.

Feeding others is also linked to identity. The role of the spouse as food preparer and/or feeder in a relationship before illness is seen in many cultures and groups. Thus, when an illness robs people of activities involving food it is not just the patient who is denied enjoyment and important experiences. The impact of cancer was studied in an urban American Chinese population where food and meals are a strong cultural indicator. Spouses and significant others were asked for their thoughts on the impact of the cancer and its treatment on their lives (Bell, Lee, & Ristovski-Slijepcevic, 2009). One person described the impact of the cancer as causing a double loss: that of the loved partner *and* of her role of being able to care and feed her loved one.

Socialization

Central to the roles that food and mealtimes play in cultures is the concept of socialization of children. At mealtimes, families teach children about roles within the family, specific practices in relation to food, and about the wider society the children live in. Across cultures, mealtimes are used as a vehicle for teaching the rules and for children to learn about the society they live in and the language that is used (Ochs & Shohet, 2006).

Meals are a time for talking about the events of the day, modelling behaviour, examining the behaviour of others, and allowing children to learn about the social, moral and behavioural rules of their society. Children learn how to be members of their own society through 'apprenticeship', i.e., copying modelled behaviour, and through language and learning about what is acceptable societal communication (De Geer, 2004; Ochs & Shohet, 2006).

Class

Class, food and mealtimes are inherently connected (Barthes, 2013; Bourdieu, 2013). There are long and detailed discussion about *class* – how it is defined, what it is and even whether it exists – which lie outside of our remit. For the purpose of this discussion, the majority of the literature refers to gross distinctions between working and middle class. Different aspirations and behaviours have been displayed by the working and middle classes (Wills, Backett-Milburn, Roberts, & Lawton, 2011).

The working class valued autonomy in food and healthy eating, aiming for their children to be able to be independent in getting, preparing and eating their food so that other tasks could then be undertaken. In contrast, the middle-class families valued the ability to eat a variety of foods, with healthy foods and exotic foods being particularly important, alongside the ability to eating with 'outsiders' and, for example, in restaurants (Wills et al., 2011).

Evidence from this work supports the existence of what might be thought of as stereotypical behaviours and beliefs. There was no difference in the financial implications of each pattern of behaviour, suggesting that the behaviours were driven by choices and aspirations rather than by money (Wills et al., 2011).

Religion

In religious contexts, food behaviours can be a core tenet. Mintz and Du Bois (2002) describe how "rituals and beliefs surrounding food can powerfully reinforce religious and ethnic boundaries" (Mintz & Du Bois, 2002, p. 107). These beliefs are often about cycles of life, the interdependence of life, and avoiding doing harm to other creatures. This is of particular importance in religions such as Buddhism and Hinduism, where behaviour in this life is believed to influence that in future lives.

Most spiritual and religious observance is intimately linked with food and mealtimes, including fasting and feasting, the special preparation of food, and the avoidance of, or abstinence from, certain foods and drinks. Fasting is common across religions, for example during Jewish Yom Kippur and Islamic Ramadan. Buddhists use a variety of methods of fasting depending on their lifestyles and requirements. Buddhists who live and work in the community may only eat before noon for six days in a month, some may remove meat from their diet (if they eat meat) for six days in a month. Buddhists monks may undertake stricter fasting periods, taking only water for up to 18 days. This is done under supervision to ensure the monk does not become ill. All fasting is undertaken by Buddhists for a range of reasons – to display consideration of those in the world suffering starvation, to ensure they are taking food only in moderation because food is meant to nourish a healthy body, to avoid over- or under-eating and to facilitate meditation. Many religions abstain from animal products, alcohol or caffeine either completely or for a defined period. Some religions require that food is slaughtered and prepared in particular ways, e.g., Halal food for Muslims and Kosher food for Jews. Halal is a way of living one's life and means 'permissible' or 'lawful'. When eating 'according to the way of Allah', eating may be a form of worship.

Most religions have times of feasting where food is consumed to mark and celebrate religious festivals. Most Christians celebrate Christmas and Easter with feasting, as do Jews at Rosh Hashanah and Passover, Buddhists for the birth, enlightenment and death of Buddha. Rastafarian meetings often include feasting on herbs of the field or land, i.e., vegetables. The taking of bread and wine is the symbolic centre of the communion sacrament for some Christians.

Cultural observances with food are important to manage within a developing disease. Increasing dysphagic symptoms may affect participation in religious festivals (Rourke & Leslie, 2013). Patients may change their mind about certain ritual observances but lack the communicative ability to explain this, or cognitive decline may result in individuals becoming less aware of religious festivals and their corresponding food rituals. These scenarios cause much anxiety for family members who remember what their loved one *used to find* important and now is not able to participate in that way, or that the observances are important to the family member themselves – a personal bias in what we feel is right or wrong.

Throughout this chapter we have discussed issues such as identity, gender, class, culture and religion. The primary purpose of presenting these issues is for us to consider how they may factor into the decision making that our patients and families have to deal with. It is important to reflect on the fact that clinicians are human beings too, and are situated in their own cultural, gendered and class contexts, with their own identities based on unique value systems. As clinicians, we need to identify our own values and biases in order to ensure that we understand how they influence our practice and beliefs. We need to be explicit about this with ourselves because our values and beliefs influence how we view our patients: *value tinted glasses*, if you like. Our world view may not fit with the patient and their views. It is important not to make any assumptions about the patient's world and their own life experiences. Clinicians must acknowledge their own biases first in order to factor them in (or out) when talking to the patient and their family. This will help to determine what is important to our patients and their lives and support robust clinical decision making.

How is this relevant to decisions in dysphagia?

Geethu-Joseph's stroke has left her with a marked right sided paralysis that has also affected her facial muscles. She is unable to walk unaided, she has significant difficulties with her speech, and she has an impaired swallow. She has also experienced some cognitive impairment – she has some memory loss and some comprehension difficulties. She is no longer able to cook for her children or her grandchildren. She finds this extremely upsetting because, up until this point, she was known for her culinary skills and she spent a lot of time looking after her grandchildren. Geethu-Joseph's difficulties following the stroke mean that she is no longer able to undertake her family tasks. This has had a serious impact on her identity and her feelings of self worth.

Her daughter-in-law now has to prepare many of the family meals which is difficult for her because she is an inexperienced cook. Due to Geethu-Joseph's physical weakness her daughter-in-law has to feed her for most meals, especially when she is tired. She can manage soft finger foods herself, but needs support with foods that require utensils. These changes have created a great deal of stress and tension within the family as finger foods and soft foods look like baby foods and to treat an elder as a child is disrespectful.

Multidisciplinary team intervention will need to acknowledge Geethu-Joseph's feelings of loss, sadness, and frustration as well as addressing her physical eating and drinking difficulties in order to be effective. It will also be important to work closely with her daughter-in-law and possibly other family members to find solutions that fit for everyone and work towards a sense of normality for the family.

David identifies closely with food, from a general interest such as growing vegetables and cooking for dinner parties, to the deeply significant cultural aspects that food and its preparation mean for his faith. He used to find great joy and meaning in family and congregational gatherings during the major Jewish religious festivals. On some occasions such as Yom Kippur, there is reflection and abstinence and on others there is much historical and religious significance in the foods that are eaten, for example the Passover Seder.

David finds himself torn; physical aspects such as nausea make him not want to even think about food but then he suffers resulting isolation from important and meaningful experiences. As time passes he knows that the mechanics of his swallow will cease to work effectively. In most religions the dietary observances may take second place to health and treating illness. David has discussed this with his Rabbi but religious permission cannot change the loss that David feels in many areas of his life regarding food and eating.

It may be beneficial for David to spend time talking about his feelings about food with his health practitioners as well as his family, his Rabbi and others. There may be alternative foods or symbolic acts that David can undertake to maintain his sense of community although this will not necessarily ease his feelings of loss regarding food and eating. In our clinical training about dysphagia, we have been steered to think about the clinical function of food, and the mechanics of the swallow, what has gone wrong with the swallow and why. We have not been guided to think about the social and individualized functions of food. We propose that not considering these means that our intervention often does not address the whole issue and is therefore unsuccessful. We have described some of the important ways in which food is central to our daily lives. Once dysphagia is an issue, either for us or for a loved family member or friend, none of the importance of the social and human acts of eating and drinking go away. Our advice to the clinician is that your clinical assessment of the swallow and formulation of a treatment plan is important. Equally central is a discussion with the patient and his/her family about what food means to them, how they feel about food, what rituals and routines are important, and who does what in relation to food within the family.

Traditional dysphagia textbooks rarely address these factors. We would argue that we cannot hope to offer person-centred, appropriate assessments or interventions without considering our patients' difficulties in their broader world perspective. We do not offer definitive *care pathways* but instead we offer a warning to recognize that there are many factors associated with food and mealtimes which may be important to the individual. Rather than making assumptions based on and biased by our own values and beliefs we must make an effort to understand the world of our patients and make recommendations that fit this world.

References

Anving, T. & Thorsted, S. (2010). Feeding ideals and the work of feeding in Swedish families: Interactions between mothers and children around the dinner table. *Food Culture & Society, 13*(1), 29-46.

Barthes, R. (2013). Towards a psychosociology of contemporary food consumption. In C. Counihan & P. Van Esterik (Eds), *Food and Culture: A Reader* (3rd ed., pp. 23-30). New York: Routledge.

Bell, K., Lee, J., & Ristovski-Slijepcevic, S. (2009). Perceptions of food and eating among Chinese patients with cancer: Findings of an ethnographic study. *Cancer Nursing, 32*(2), 118-126.

Bourdieu, P. (2013). Distinction: A social critique of the judgement of taste (R. Nice, Trans.). In C. Counihan & P. Van Esterik (Eds), *Food and Culture: A Reader* (3rd ed., pp. 31-39). New York: Routledge.

Bugge, A.B. & Almås, R. (2006). Domestic dinner: Representations and practices of a proper meal among young suburban mothers. *Journal of Consumer Culture, 6*(2), 203-228.

Carrington, C. (1999). *No Place Like Home: Relationships and Family Life among Lesbians and Gay Men.* Chicago: University of Chicago Press.

Cason, K.L. (2006). Family mealtimes: More than just eating together. *Journal of the American Dietetic Association, 106*(4), 532-533.

Charles, N. & Kerr, M. (1988). *Women, Food, and Families.* Manchester, UK; New York: Manchester University Press. Distributed exclusively in the USA and Canada by St. Martin's Press.

D'Sylva, A. & Beagan, B.L. (2011). 'Food is culture, but it's also power': The role of food in ethnic and gender identity construction among Goan Canadian women. *Journal of Gender Studies, 20*(3), 279-289.

De Geer, B. (2004). "Don't say it's disgusting!" Comments on socio-moral behavior in Swedish families. *Journal of Pragmatics, 36*(9), 1705-1725.

DeVault, M.L. (1991). *Feeding the Family: The Social Organization of Caring as Gendered Work.* Chicago: University of Chicago Press.

Fiese, B.H., Foley, K.P., & Spagnola, M. (2006). Routine and ritual elements in family mealtimes: Contexts for child well-being and family identity. *New Directions in Child Adolescent Development,* 111, 67-89.

Fjellström, C. (2008). Mealtime and meal patterns from a cultural perspective. *Scandinavian Journal of Nutrition, 48*(4), 4.

Grieshaber, S. (1997). Mealtime rituals: Power and resistance in the construction of mealtime rules. *British Journal of Sociology, 48*(4), 649-666.

Hocking, C., Wright-St. Clair, V., & Bunrayong, W. (2002). The meaning of cooking and recipe work for older Thai and New Zealand women. *Journal of Occupational Science, 9*(3), 117-127.

Meah, A. (2014). Reconceptualizing power and gendered subjectivities in domestic cooking spaces. *Progress in Human Geography, 38*(5), 671-690.

Miller, L., Rozin, P., & Fiske, A.P. (1998). Food sharing and feeding another person suggest intimacy: Two studies of American college students. *European Journal of Social Psychology, 28*(3), 423-436.

Mintz, S.W. & Du Bois, C.M. (2002). The anthropology of food and eating. *Annual Review of Anthropology, 31*, 99-119.

Moisio, R., Arnould, E.J., & Price, L.L. (2004). Between mothers and markets: Constructing family identity through homemade food. *Journal of Consumer Culture, 4*(3), 361-384.

Neumark-Sztainer, D., Hannan, P.J., Story, M., Croll, J., & Perry, C. (2003). Family meal patterns: Associations with sociodemographic characteristics and improved dietary intake among adolescents. *Journal of the American Dietetic Association, 103*(3), 317-322.

Neumark-Sztainer, D., Story, M., Ackard, D., Moe, J., & Perry, C. (2000). The "family meal": Views of adolescents. *Journal of Nutrition Education, 32*(6), 329-334.

Ochs, E. & Shohet, M. (2006). The cultural structuring of mealtime socialization. *New Directions in Child Adolescent Development,* 111, 35-49.

Pan, W.H., Hsieh, Y.T., & Wahlqvist, M.L. (2009). Gender-specific roles and needs in food-health security. *Asia Pacific Journal of Clinical Nutrition, 18*(4), 642-646.

Rourke, N. & Leslie, P. (2003). Sacremental swallow: How swallowing informs eucharistic theology. *National Catholic Bioethics Quarterley, 13* (2), 253 – 262.

Warde, A. & Hetherington, K. (1994). English households and routine food practices - A Research Note. *Sociological Review, 42*(4), 758-778.

Warin, M., Turner, K., Moore, V., & Davies, M. (2008). Bodies, mothers and identities: Rethinking obesity and the BMI. *Sociology of Health & Illness, 30*(1), 97-111.

Wilk, R.R. (1999). "Real Belizean food": Building local identity in the transnational caribbean. *American Anthropologist, 101*(2), 244-255.

Wills, W., Backett-Milburn, K., Roberts, M.L., & Lawton, J. (2011). The framing of social class distinctions through family food and eating practices. *Sociological Review, 59*(4), 725-740.

3 Bioethics, informed consent and disclosure

Decision making around food and feeding is never thought about until there is a problem. Typical problems may be, for example, restrictions on certain types of food (low sodium diets), drastic physical reactions (shellfish allergy), route of intake (feeding tubes after oral surgery), or consistency (no solid food). Clinicians sometimes find themselves in a battle of wills over professional advice. This is perhaps more distressing because of the grey nature of the issues: rarely absolutely good or bad, rarely immediately threatening to life, or guaranteeing improvement. More knowledge about the biochemistry of the food, or details of cortical swallowing control is possible but we propose that substantive help lies in a different direction. Let us consider our decision making from a different perspective than the facts and diagnostic or intervention approach from our clinical education. We turn in this chapter to the discipline of bioethics. We will also review what is meant by *informed consent* and some foundational legal work.

The rise of 'bioethics'

This book is not a philosophy or bioethics text, so a detailed examination of theory is beyond our remit. A consideration of the history of bioethics and some concepts from philosophy and ethics will help us understand the points of view of others with whom we might interact during decision making. These topics are also useful for framing our deliberations. Bioethics is the area of ethical study concerned with issues in healthcare, life sciences and clinical research. A good question to ask is how scientific questions (research) are different to bioethical questions:

> "The major difference between bioethical and scientific inquiry is that scientists seek to understand phenomena in the world - they want to describe what is - while bioethicists seek to figure out what people should do."
>
> National Institute for Health, 2009

What *should* we do? This is the perennial clinical question.

What is 'bioethics'?

The role of bioethics may be thought of as using ethical concepts to help clinicians, and more broadly policymakers and researchers, make decisions.

> "You probably faced a clinical issue today with an ethical component. Did you recognize it…? Did you know what to do?"
>
> Singer & Viens, 2008, p. 1

According to *The Cambridge Textbook of Bioethics*, 'bioethics' is firmly placed in the real clinical world of healthcare professionals and patients (Singer & Viens, 2008). Improving patient care by developing clinicians' knowledge of bioethical issues requires input from such diverse fields as philosophy, law, politics, biotechnology and religion. Deciding which antibiotic to use might be a purely clinical question based on the strain of bacteria: Fred has a throat infection where antibiotic A is known to work and the bacteria is resistant to antibiotic B. But say Fred is a surgeon with a wound infection that might lead to amputation of his dominant arm. And preterm baby Enid has an infection that might lead to profound deafness. The pharmacy only has enough of the antibiotic to treat one of these patients – how do we decide on this?

Bioethics is an active process: case to theory to case to theory, rather than just the application of some theoretical principles to a case in a one-way fashion. *Hypothesis led intervention* is how most clinicians are educated: we predict what might be going on based on some data, we try a treatment based on our hypothesis, and then we review our predictions and amend intervention as necessary. Both of these approaches are iterative and allow for improvement in approach presuming we reflect as we go along. Professionals are required to reflect on their own actions, on the situation and on how others might act. This reflection helps to make externally validated and reasonable decisions. External validation comes from communicating with other disciplines and results in more 'informed' decisions.

What is the subject matter of bioethics?

When we think about bioethics it is often in relation to traditional hot topics such as end of life care, pregnant women and unborn foetus rights, genetics, and biotechnology. The question of how to approach matters in practice finds bioethicists attempting to answer the *yes but so what* question that people often ask following well-meaning advice or theory. Any member of a clinical email list will be familiar with topics such as advance directives, did Patient X have the capacity to make that decision, should I withdraw care when my patient refuses to follow my advice? Most of these problems arise because of *inadequate communication* rather than dramatic moral conundrums (Leslie & Casper, 2015). We propose that a knowledge of bioethics is suited to the clinical world of swallow problems and indeed may well help us to address our *grey* areas.

Who is a bioethicist?

Bioethics is about improving the patient (and family) experience; thus, a 'bioethicist' may be a formally trained specialist in bioethics or a clinician in a relationship with the patient (or their family). There is no *one* discipline that could or should make all the bioethical decisions. The field is about people who have insight into more than one discipline whether they come from a legal background with training in clinical ethics, or a clinician with training in law and philosophy. People do not have to be formally educated experts but should have familiarity with other perspectives and approaches. Any individual pondering the bioethics of a situation must look outward for information to bring back to bear on the case or issue at hand.

Multidisciplinary work was the direction in which healthcare moved in the latter part of the 20th century. This acknowledged that there was more than one facet to a patient's illness and life. In the last two decades, a further move has been made to try to address the nebulous, conscience nagging, ethically grey areas that surface in real healthcare. Thus, clinicians need to consider the ethical view of their patients' care and those outside of the clinical discipline.

Whose bioethics?

There are more interests that must be served than an individual's own. Most bioethics and clinical texts advocate that there are different perspectives and cultures which should be respected. It is a person's *relationship* with his or her religion that is crucial rather than, say, whether they are Roman Catholic. It is not simply a matter of a direct translation from one system to another. Different cultures may view health, illness and ethics in a conceptually and structurally different way. For example, the principle of autonomy is viewed as a very individually centred concept in most western cultures. In many eastern cultures the locus of autonomy is that of the family or societal group. When we are trying to work through a clinical and bioethical problem we should use reasoned judgement taking the case *and the context* into consideration. The 'right' decision, or more likely the 'least bad' one, will depend upon the lens through which it is viewed. So for a patient the preferred outcome might be independence but for the clinician that might represent increased risk of something bad happening.

The world had *ethics* and *scientific progress* for at least 2000 years without *bioethics*. Bioethics encourages us to look at the complexity of a decision and think **whose** perspective is driving this? We therefore appreciate that the human at the centre of the difficult decision making process is important and not just their larynx, and that there are connections between that single person, their family, the healthcare institute and society. Likewise, those connections will influence the specific decision regarding impairment or treatments involving said larynx. Case by case reasoned clinical judgement with external validation from such a range of disciplines is a useful construct of bioethics.

Informed consent

In medicine, the principle of asking a patient to give permission for an intervention to be performed on him or her has been well established over the last century. This is known as obtaining consent and for it to be legally defensible it must be *informed* consent. This requires that clinicians share information with patients and families to help with decision making. Informed consent is a process by which decision makers should be walked through the treatment options, including that of no treatment, by the responsible clinician. This requires *disclosure* of information by the clinician. A risk analysis of possible costs and benefits should be undertaken so that the patient can make a knowledgeable (*informed*) decision to permit (*consent*) the clinician to undertake the intervention.

National physician bodies such as the General Medical Council (GMC, UK) and the American Medical Association (AMA, USA) acknowledge that informed consent should be a process involving discussion between the healthcare provider and patient (or family). The GMC advises:

- Listen to patients and respect their views about their health

- Discuss with patients what their diagnosis, prognosis, treatment and care involve

- Share with patients the information they want or need in order to make decisions

- Maximize patients' opportunities, and their ability, to make decisions for themselves

- Respect patients' decisions.

(GMC, 2016a)

The AMA requires that physicians provide:

- Disclosure and discussion (risks, benefits, no treatment, diagnosis, etc.)

- An opportunity for the patient to ask questions to better understand options.

(AMA, 2006, 2013)

We include these physician codes because they reflect what any clinician should ensure with their patients. Unfortunately, the *process* of informed consent became an *event* ("did you consent the patient"). At its worst, this means, did you get a signature on some form that purports to absolve the health care provider of legal liability (Lidz, Appelbaum, & Meisel, 1988).

In the UK, the Health and Care Professions Council (HCPC) states that all registrants must, among other responsibilities:

"1. Promote and protect the interests of service users and carers

1.4 You must make sure that you have consent from service users or other appropriate authority before you provide care, treatment or other services

2. Communicate appropriately and effectively."

(Health & Care Professions Council, 2016, pp. 5-6)

The Royal College of Speech and Language Therapists has an open access webpage containing a number of resources regarding consent to treatment and issues such as video or audio recording (The Royal College of Speech and Language Therapists, 2016).

What is adequate disclosure?

For a patient to give permission for a physician to treat them has been a legal concept in the UK since the late 18th century (Mazur, 2003).The idea that a physician had a responsibility to inform a patient of *possible consequences* of treatment *before* the patient gave such permission was not really clearly voiced in the legal world until the mid-20th century with the California case of Salgo v. Leland ("Salgo v. Leland Stanford Jr University Board of Trustees," 1957). Gradually, the principle was established that a physician must gain *informed* consent or face a charge of professional negligence, and thus a 'standard of disclosure' came into being as part of reasonable professional practice.

But what exactly must a physician disclose? In 1972, the Canterbury v. Spence case moved us towards a consideration of what is *material* to the patient ("Canterbury v. Spence," 1972). In order to make a decision, we need information about how the options *might work for us*. This move to increase the information disclosed and make it specific to a patient seemed to be wise: not just a standard for a professional to disclose but a standard based on a patient's needs.

What conditions are required?

For a decision to be made and informed consent given, the decision maker must be acting autonomously. What circumstances do we need for this? Across the varying disciplines concerned with *autonomy* we consistently see that three conditions are required (Beauchamp & Childress, 1994):

- **Intentionality**: "I intend to do this thing. I am choosing the pudding rather than the soup on my tray because I prefer it and not because I have a hemianopia and I *cannot see* the soup on the left of my table."

- **Understanding**: "I understand what is involved in the different courses of action. This requires that I can weigh up the costs and benefits of the outcomes. A way to assess this is for a person to 'teach back' the rationale, i.e., explain back to the clinician why they pick a certain course of action over others."

- **Voluntariness**: "I am making my choice without coercion. As clinicians, we would be horrified to think that we were *coercing* a patient or family member. But there are subtle forces at play: the clinician-patient relationship is not an equal one no matter how much effort a clinician puts in to this. Patients often want to please their healthcare providers or fear that if they disagree or report failure that the clinician will be disappointed or worse – take retribution."

Following on from these requirements for autonomy is the need for a person to be able to communicate their wishes. Even if someone can understand the options, costs, benefits and consequences they cannot give consent if they cannot communicate their wishes (Appelbaum & Grisso, 1988; Sharp, 2015). Thus the role of professionals who work with patients who have communication disorders is doubly important: we are involved with difficult decisions regarding eating and drinking that have to be made by people with impaired communication.

Fluctuating capacity

Of course, many of our patients do not have a constant degree of capacity or incapacity, it fluctuates throughout the day or when their health or emotional status deteriorates or improves. The same can be said for anyone: capacity is for a *particular decision* at a *particular moment in time*. So we understand that a single parent with two small children and no support network, who has just been given a diagnosis of an incurable aggressive cancer, should not be asked about experimental treatments because they are processing the dreadful news. As far as possible, clinicians must act to make the decision understandable to the person involved and not simply presume that anyone cannot understand matters. Defence of a robust decision making process will be seen in the documentation of the discussion, who said what to whom. We just have to be seen to have tried our best. We might start with simple steps:

- Have the discussion(s) when the person is most alert in the day

- Be mindful of other issues that they are thinking about

- Align with the medication schedule to optimize the ability to process information

- Use diagrams or pictures.

These will help us align with the requirements for legal competence:

- Communicating a choice

- Understanding relevant information

- Appreciating the current situation and its consequences

- Manipulating information rationally.

(Appelbaum & Grisso, 1988)

There is increasing evidence that people with cognitive impairments need careful assessment of their decisional capacity which often is greater than has been historically presumed (Karlawish, 2008). For people at risk of lacking capacity there are many factors that play into the decision making but institutions and countries' legal systems are developing structures to support this (Clarke, Galbraith, Woodward, Holland, & Barclay, 2015).

Legal considerations

Both the UK and USA have case-based (case or tort) law and broader reaching legislation. This is not a comprehensive legal text but there are certain concepts that have been addressed in both legal systems. As previously mentioned, there are seminal cases in the USA such as the Salgo and Canterbury cases.

In the UK, people may be familiar with cases such as Case MB in 1997 which determined that capacity relates to that instance in time and that particular decision. Case B in 2002 established that a patient can refuse treatment even if it results in death and clinicians must respect that decision. Equally, clinicians (specifically in this case physicians) are under no legal obligation to provide a treatment that is futile (GMC, 2016b). Legislation is further reaching than case law but is a much bigger undertaking to get established. A clinician has to be clear what applies to their particular work setting and location. We will consider examples from the UK and USA.

UK: Capacity type acts

In 2002, the Adults with Incapacity Act (Scotland) came into being. It addressed the need to safeguard the welfare of people over the age of consent (16 years) who are deemed to be without decisional capacity due to impaired mental status/communication ability (Mental Welfare Commission for Scotland, 2000). The Act provides guidance regarding the necessity of the intervention (including healthcare) and what surrogate decision makers must take into account. Surrogate decision makers must also demonstrate that the patient was actively encouraged to use whatever skills they had to participate in the process.

In 2005, the Mental Capacity Act (England and Wales) set out that adults must be presumed to have capacity until proven otherwise, and that this must follow only after all reasonable attempts have been made to help the person make the decision (Office of the Public Guardian, 2005). Each health practitioner responsible for a particular assessment or intervention is responsible for determining whether patients under their care understand their treatment. In order to make a decision, an individual must be able to understand, retain and use relevant information to make their own decision. They also must be able to communicate their decision.

USA: Standards of disclosure and federal legislation

What information should be shared (physician disclosure) falls under two standards: the **reasonable physician standard** and the **reasonable patient standard**. The reasonable physician standard compares a physician's actions to that of his professional peers. This makes commonsense: that a professional is acting within the scope and manner of the majority of his fellow practitioners. This presumes that the majority is acting in an appropriate manner, with up-to-date practice, and aligned with current clinical guidelines.

The reasonable patient standard accepts that *what needs to be discussed* should map to *what the patient needs to know* in order to select a treatment, or no treatment. This also makes sense. As patients, we lean towards the idea that we want all the information that is material to us. The problem is that it is impossible to know exactly what is material. Clinical professionals looking to follow the 'rules' from the outset struggle to find clear guidelines on what 'reasonable' really means. We propose this requires an ongoing dialogue with the patient, family and other members of the clinical team.

In the USA, legislation is harder to enact given the legal system and state authority but 27 years ago an Act was passed that is still highly relevant today. In 1990, the Patient Self Determination Act was passed to ensure that patients were informed that they had a right to make advance directives and that they could state to accept *or refuse* medical care ("Patient Self Determination Act," 1990). Organizations participating in federal reimbursement schemes such as **Medicare** (the insurance programme for people who are aged 65 years or older, certain younger people with disabilities, and people with end-stage renal disease) and **Medicaid** (limited provision for people with low income and restricted resources) are required to address advance directive issues and acceptance or refusal of care with patients. The right to accept or refuse medical care is not restricted to the end-of-life decisions that we typically associate with advance directives. In 1914, in the case of Schloendorff v. Society of New York Hospital, Justice Cardozo summed up this legal position:

> "Every human being of adult years and sound mind has a right to determine what shall be done with his own body and cannot be subjected to medical treatment without his consent"
>
> ("Schloendorff v. Society of New York Hospital," 1914)

This is a foundational principle in many countries even today.

How is this relevant to decisions in dysphagia?

David is having increasing difficulties with eating and drinking and the clinical team have raised the idea of a gastrostomy feeding tube. David's wife, Abigail, is very supportive of this option and so was devastated when David announced that he was going to decline the intervention. Abigail and some of the clinical staff have questioned David's capacity to make this decision, citing possible effects of the cancer treatment or the pain medications.

Understanding legal and ethical issues surrounding capacity is extremely important when working in any clinical area, but particularly when patients are making difficult decisions about food. As we have discussed, food is not just a biological, / medical intervention, it intersects with many areas of our lives and impacts on our emotional, physical and psychological wellbeing. It is interesting how people usually only question another's capacity when there is disagreement rather than agreement. Further exploration of Abigail's perspective reveals that she is not ready to accept that David is dying and that, as she sees it, her time with him will be cut short by his choice. As deeply sad as this is, we must respect David's wishes after ensuring that he understands the possible benefits and costs of the tube option and of no tube option. Many patients agree to treatment because they know how much their family members want it and we must draw out each person's views, possibly separately. Part of our role is in education and even mediation between family members.

Nan has always enjoyed her monthly visits with her sister. During these visits, they go to the theatre where Nan often has a gin and tonic and some peanuts. She particularly enjoys this part of the visit. Recently, she has begun to cough on the nuts. Nan's sister feels this is an important part of the visit and that Nan has the capacity to understand that the nuts make her cough but that she still wants to go ahead and have them. The staff in the home feel that Nan does not have the capacity to make a decision about the nuts and that it would be in her best interests not to have any further nuts because of the coughing. They are also concerned about the risk of choking on the nuts, although so far this has not been observed.

As the clinician responsible for assessing Nan's eating and drinking skills it will be important for us to determine Nan's level of understanding of all the issues associated with eating the perceived high-risk food, alongside her actual ability to undertake this activity. It is important to think broadly about the activity, and to talk with Nan and her family about the activity and negotiate which parts can be changed and which are essential in order for Nan to enjoy the outing. It may be determined that Nan has the capacity to understand the risks, and we may need to support her in her chosen route even if this is not the healthcare professional's ideal choice. It may be that she does not have capacity to understand the issues. In this case, we must still support Nan to undertake her chosen activity in a way that honours her wishes should she have been able to articulate them, but that also considers her safety and best interests. Best interests should be discussed with reference to Nan's wishes, those of her family and friends, and the multidisciplinary team working with Nan. Whether she has capacity or not, Nan has clearly indicated she thoroughly enjoys the nuts, so every effort must be made to replicate this experience as closely as possible.

References

AMA. (2006). Opinion 8.08 - Informed Consent. Retrieved 1 March 2013, from http://www.ama-assn.org/ama/pub/physician-resources/medical-ethics/code-medical-ethics/opinion808.page

AMA. (2013). Informed Consent. Retrieved 1 March 2013, from http://www.ama-assn.org/ama/pub/physician-resources/legal-topics/patient-physician-relationship-topics/informed-consent.page

Appelbaum, P.S. & Grisso, T. (1988). Assessing patients' capacities to consent to treatment. *New England Journal of Medicine, 319*(25), 1635-1638.

Beauchamp, T. & Childress, J. (1994). *Principles of Biomedical Ethics* (4th ed.). Oxford: Oxford University Press.

Canterbury v. Spence, 464 F.2d 772 (150 U.S.App.D.C. 263 1972).

Clarke, G., Galbraith, S., Woodward, J., Holland, A., & Barclay, S. (2015). Eating and drinking interventions for people at risk of lacking decision-making capacity: Who decides and how? *BMC Medical Ethics, 16*, 41.

GMC. (2016a). Consent Guidance: Part 1: Principles. *Good Medical Practice.* Retrieved 22 May 2016, from http://www.gmc-uk.org/guidance/ethical_guidance/consent_guidance_part1_principles.asp

GMC. (2016b). End of Life Care: Legal Annex. *Good Medical Practice*. Retrieved 22 May 2016, from http://www.gmc-uk.org/guidance/ethical_guidance/end_of_life_legal_annex.asp

Health & Care Professions Council. (2016). Your duties as a registrant: Standards of conduct, performance and ethics. (20120801POLPUB/SCPE (updated January 2016)). London: Health & Care Professions Council. Retrieved from http://www.hcpc-uk.org/assets/do cuments/10004EDFStandardsofconduct,performanceandethics.pdf.

Karlawish, J. (2008). Measuring decision-making capacity in cognitively impaired individuals. *Neurosignals, 16*(1), 91–98.

Leslie, P. & Casper, M. (2015). Ethical challenges: Less about moral wrongdoing and more about communication breakdown. *SIG 15 Perspectives on Gerontology, 20*(3), 72–84.

Lidz, C.W., Appelbaum, P.S., & Meisel, A. (1988). Two models of implementing informed consent. *Archives of Internal Medicine, 148*(6), 1385–1389.

Mazur, D. (2003). Influence of the law on risk and informed consent. *BMJ, 327*(7417), 731–734.

Mental Welfare Commission for Scotland. (2000). Adults with Incapacity (Scotland) Act. Retrieved 25 June 2016, from http://www.mwcscot.org.uk/the-law/adults-with-incapacity-act/

National Institutes for Health. (2009). Teaching Exploring Bioethics. Retrieved 31 May 2016, from https://science.education.nih.gov/supplements/nih9/bioethics/guide/pdf/ Teachers_Guide.pdf

Office of the Public Guardian. (2005, 22 October 2014). Mental Capacity Act. Retrieved 26 May 2016, from https://www.justice.gov.uk/protecting-the-vulnerable/mental-capacity-act

Patient Self Determination Act, 42 U.S.C. § 1395cc (a) (1) (1990).

Salgo v. Leland Stanford Jr University Board of Trustees, 317 P2d 170 (154 Cal App2d 560 1957).

Schloendorff v. Society of New York Hospital, 105 N.E. 92 (211 NY 125 1914).

Sharp, H.M. (2015). Informed consent in clinical and research settings: What do patients and families need to make informed decisions? *SIG 13 Perspectives on Swallowing and Swallowing Disorders (Dysphagia), 24*(4), 130–139.

Singer, P.A. & Viens, A.M. (2008). *The Cambridge Textbook of Bioethics*. Cambridge; New York: Cambridge University Press.

The Royal College of Speech and Language Therapists. (2016). Information Governance: Consent. Retrieved 25 June 2016, from https://www.rcslt.org/cq_live/resources_a_z/ info_gov/consent

4 Families

This chapter addresses some of the issues that may arise for family carers when caring for a loved one with dysphagia. It is really important that we think about working closely and carefully with family carers because they are often intimately involved with supporting their loved ones on a day-to-day basis and they may have to make treatment decisions if their loved ones lack the capacity to make decisions for themselves. Family carers are often the ones who have to implement our recommendations. Where intervention is long term we need to consider how recommendations may affect the lives of patients and their loved ones.

When we ask families to be involved in decisions on behalf of their loved ones they may feel overwhelmed due to the complexity of the decision and it being required at a time when family carers are themselves under stress. Again and again we come up against cases involving people with dysphagia, but some feel much more difficult to manage than others. We have never been able to come up with a formula or flow diagram for assessing, managing and treating dysphagia – why is this? It is because each individual patient case is unique. Each patient has a life story, likes, dislikes, and preferences. Each patient has a unique set of people around them, and each is embedded within a culture and a set of beliefs. So is there any wonder that we struggle to come up with a formula that advises clinicians how to manage dysphagia? If we examine some of the issues that may stress family carers, we can then consider this in the context of decision making.

Family carer stress

When we work with family carers who are required to engage in decision making on behalf of their loved one, it is important to think about factors that cause stress. If we do not understand the context that our patients and their families live in, then we may fail to support them appropriately. Decisions that surrogates make on behalf of another will affect the decision maker and the patient's wider network as well as the patient. It may be that a valued activity such as going out to eat in a restaurant is no longer possible. Or a family carer has to start preparing all meals after years of it being their loved one's role. Making recommendations to permanently change what people eat and how they eat also influences the activities associated with eating and drinking. It is very rare that a practitioner talking with a family member in June will think to ask, "and how might this affect Christmas day, and how can we help you to still make that a good day?"

Families may be experiencing increased burdens associated with other aspects of their loved one's illness (O'Reilly, Finnan, Allwright, Smith, & Ben-Shlomo, 1996). Stress and burden depend on several factors such as the degree of physical care, poor carer/patient relationship, patient's incontinence, financial consequences and lack of support for the family carer (Pochard et al., 2005). Each individual stress factor creates a burden and there is an interaction effect akin to polypharmacy where each drug has side effects but they also interact with each other in an unpredictable way and cause more problems. *Psychological and physical malaise* is a phrase used to describe the consequences of caring experienced by the carer (Nolan, Grant, & Ellis, 1990).

Stress factors

There is increasing evidence that families caring for a sick loved one will be under a significant amount of pressure. Family carers suffer physically, psychologically, and in terms of their own health habits (Schulz & Sherwood, 2008). There is evidence to suggest that whether their loved one is experiencing a chronic long-term illness, or has had a recent acute illness, family carers suffer from depression, anxiety, financial hardship and have poor health outcomes (Pochard et al., 2005; Vitaliano, Zhang, & Scanlan, 2003). Family carers who experience such pressures may find it difficult to participate in decision making on behalf of their loved one (Whitlatch, 2008). At the point when decisions need to be made, families are often out of their usual environment, possibly sleep deprived and may be feeling a range of emotions, such as anxiety, anger, and/or guilt. This stress on family carers may be long-term and chronic. As part of our intervention we must understand the family carers' perspective and stress as well as our patient's. We have a duty to ensure that we work with family carers in a way that takes account of their stress, their priorities and their beliefs (Health & Care Professions Council, 2016).

There are occasions when lengthy consultation with family members about medical intervention is not possible. In acute situations where life-saving intervention is required the intervention takes priority over family discussions. In such scenarios, family discussion should still be a priority as soon as possible (Flynn et al., 2012).

If we accept that family carers may be suffering psychologically then we can examine the type of things that cause families pressure and stress. This is particularly important if a loved one has recently become ill and the diagnosis or prognosis may have been a shock. In residential care or acute settings, family carers may suffer stress if their loved one is sharing a room with other patients. If the patient is at home and chronically unwell, family carers may be missing out on social events or struggling with daily tasks such as shopping because they cannot leave the house. The age of the family carer and the meaning that they see in their caregiving may have an impact on the levels of stress experienced, or the care required may be physically burdensome (Haley, LaMonde, Han, Burton, & Schonwetter, 2003; Pochard et al., 2005; Stancin, Wade, Walz, Yeates, & Taylor, 2008).

When physical and cognitive difficulties are coupled with behaviour difficulties this may be particularly stressful for family carers (Lecavalier, Leone, & Wiltz, 2006). While family carers sometimes report that caring for their loved one brings them closer, it is often at the expense of other social relationships (Haley et al., 2003). Family carers may suffer from financial hardship, particularly if the patient contributed to the family income (Lai, 2012). Further costs may include travelling to visit a loved one in care, the family carer themselves having to give up work, or being unable to work in the first place because of providing care. There may be existing responsibilities to other dependents.

Relationship issues

When working with family carers we must consider the relationship between the carer, their loved one and the rest of the family. The things that stress one individual may be different to those that stress another. A parent caring for a young child with physical disabilities may be stressed by different things than an elderly man caring for his wife who has dementia. Changes in relationships due to illness may themselves be a source of stress for patients and family carers. Family carers may for the first time become the driver, the chef, the house cleaner, the planner, the budget holder, or the nurse to a patient, which was not a role expected when the relationship began. This can be extremely stressful for carers (Dekel, Solomon, & Bleich, 2005). The carer might be the spouse, parent, sibling, other relative or a close friend. Each relationship will be different and will influence family carers' thoughts and decision making. This further contributes to the interaction effect of multiple stressors (Nolan et al., 1990).

Decision making on behalf of another

Individuals' opinions and beliefs about their health develop over time. These opinions and beliefs are influenced by personal values embedded and developed within their culture, and experiences. When people become ill, they use these opinions and beliefs in decision making about their health care. When an individual loses capacity to engage in their own decision making they are unable to voice their opinions or take part in the discussion and decision making about their own care. So family carers must engage in discussion and decision making on behalf of their loved one but they also have values and beliefs which may align or not with their loved one's preferences (Moon, Townsend, Whitlatch, & Dilworth-Anderson, 2016).

Surrogates (usually) have the best interest of the patient in mind but may still be subject to unconscious bias. One study looked at decision making in real families where a decision had to be made in the near future (rather than previous hypothetical or long-term prediction work with students) on (1) heart resuscitation, and (2) extending life vs pain relief (Marks & Arkes, 2008). Where the patient and surrogate chose different options (i.e., surrogate error in prediction) the majority of surrogates chose *what they would want for the patient* rather than what they thought the patient would want. This was termed 'projection' (Marks & Arkes, 2008). We as professionals should be alert to this possibility and support family carers in working out what the patient would have wanted if they could voice their opinion.

Outcomes

There is a continual drive in healthcare to prove that the interventions we offer have successful outcomes. But what outcomes are we aiming for? It may be difficult to predict the patient's overall prognosis and therefore even more difficult to predict the prognosis in relation to dysphagia. What is a *good outcome* for an individual patient and their family? It is likely to be different for everyone depending on personal values and beliefs. Decisions to be made about assessment and intervention should be *guided* and *advised* by the health practitioner but it is important to consider whose decision it ultimately is. Decisions affect a person's health and wellbeing, the whole family's quality of life, identity, and the way they live their lives day to day.

Family carers may need encouragement to think through the range of options for their loved one, who just happens to be your patient, in order to arrive at the best fit intervention. We need to be certain that, as clinicians, we do not allow our own personal beliefs and values to bias the professional advice that we give. In a study regarding feeding tube recommendations for patients with dementia, relatively few SLTs reported expected benefit with respect to comfort, functional status, or quality of life (Sharp & Shega, 2009). But more than 50% of the same SLTs would recommend tube feeding in a patient with advanced dementia and dysphagia when a patient's preferences are unknown.

The practitioner and multidisciplinary team need to help family carers to come to the right decision *for their loved one*, and then support them in that decision. From a professional point of view the practitioner must ensure that they have provided a range of options based on the best available evidence, chosen through their own clinical experience, and with regard to their knowledge of the patient/family preferences and situation. Options should be presented in a balanced, honest and unbiased way as far as possible whilst still acknowledging that they are giving their professional opinion. Patients and family carers come to clinical specialists because they have knowledge that most people do not, so to lay out options and then say *just pick* does not support autonomy.

As a practitioner, we should offer our thoughts on the best option from our professional standpoint and then work with family carers who need to balance the options against the other factors that are of relevance to them. It is our duty to enable patients and families to ask the questions they do not even know that they need to ask. This helps family carers use information to make the right decisions for their loved one. As long as we have made sure the decision making process is robust, then you have discharged our professional duty.

How is this relevant to dysphagia?

For Henry's family, the day starts at 6am when he needs to be woken for chest percussion which takes 20 minutes. Following this, Henry has a bath and is dressed. At 8am he has his breakfast, which takes about an hour because Henry has difficulties with managing his food orally and all his food needs to be well mashed and moist. At 9am, Henry has his medication and then takes part in an activity. Henry needs to return to a base at noon to have his second session of chest percussion, his lunch, and his second dose of medication. Henry often has a nap after his lunch. He sometimes feels well enough to take part in an activity in the afternoon. He then needs to be back at home for 5pm to have his nebulizer, and then at 6pm he has more chest percussion. He has a small meal after his chest percussion from 6:30-8:00pm. He then has his medication. Henry needs to sit upright for half an hour after all meals. At 8:30pm Henry goes to bed. He usually sleeps soundly until he is woken at midnight for chest percussion. Henry is sometimes able to doze through this, and other times he wakes fully. Henry is then settled again at about 12:30am and sleeps until 6:00am. Henry needs this routine every day and support is required 24 hours a day. This means that his mother can no longer work.

Henry's difficulties and his mother's inability to work significantly impact the family finances, as his mother had a good job working as an officer manager. The change in financial circumstances is causing tension because Henry's father has to work extra shifts to support the family. Henry's two teenage sisters have also been impacted by the financial burden. Henry's mother is tired and feels 'backed into a corner' by the need to care for Henry and being in such a difficult financial position. In our management, we need to understand the context in which Henry's dysphagia is being managed. The family's report of stress, tiredness and pressure as a result of their financial circumstances is influencing their ability to focus on engaging in clinical discussions about Henry's dysphagia.

Clinicians should strive to sensitively understand the lives of the families they work with and the demands and stresses they have placed on them. This will allow more sensitive and person -centred interventions. Establishing what is uppermost in the family's mind as regards Henry and eating/drinking goals rather than the activity may help. For many the goal is to maintain health, enjoy social connections, have pleasure in tastes of favourite foods. Discussion of overall goals might open the way to the possibility of alternative routes to supplementing Henry's diet whilst maintaining pleasure feeding. Taking a step back with the family to look at fatigue, time, stress and their burden as a unit may allow for options that do not feel to the family like they are giving up on Henry and his eating.

David has begun to talk in less detail about his thoughts about his illness and treatment with Abigail. She reports that she feels 'shut out' by David. They have differing opinions about the best treatment options for his developing dysphagia. Abigail also reports that she feels less like his wife and more like his carer. She has to remind him to take his tablets, modify his food for him, and support him physically when they are out and about.

We can see here how David's illness is changing the relationship between him and his wife. It is likely that there will also be changes in his relationship with his teenage children, and that all of these may cause stress, tension and sadness. The stress of illness can lead people to disengage from social supports. It is important to observe the family relationships within a clinical setting. If positive therapeutic relationships are developed it may be possible to offer support so that families can be helped to talk about their feelings and look for solutions. Referral families for more specialist support may be discussed as part of the ongoing clinical team care approach..

In this chapter we have considered some of the sources of pressure on family carers of people with dysphagia and the importance of personal relationships informing carer decision making. When people have to make decisions on behalf of another who lacks capacity, the burden is even greater.

References

Dekel, R., Solomon, Z., & Bleich, A. (2005). Emotional distress and marital adjustment of caregivers: Contribution of level of impairment and appraised burden. *Anxiety, Stress, & Coping, 18*(1), 71-82.

Flynn, D., Knoedler, M.A., Hess, E.P., Murad, M.H., Erwin, P.J., Montori, V.M., & Thomson, R.G. (2012). Engaging patients in health care decisions in the emergency department through shared decision-making: A systematic review. *Academy of Emerging Medicine, 19*(8), 959–967.

Haley, W.E., LaMonde, L.A., Han, B., Burton, A.M., & Schonwetter, R. (2003). Predictors of depression and life satisfaction among spousal caregivers in hospice: Application of a stress process model. *Journal of Palliative Medicine, 6*(2), 215–224.

Health & Care Professions Council. (2016). Your duties as a registrant: Standards of conduct, performance and ethics. (20120801POLPUB/SCPE (updated January 2016)). London: Health & Care Professions Council. Retrieved from http://www.hcpc-uk.org/assets/do cuments/10004EDFStandardsofconduct,performanceandethics.pdf

Lai, D.W.L. (2012). Effect of financial costs on caregiving burden of family caregivers of older adults. *SAGE Open, 2*(4).

Lecavalier, L., Leone, S., & Wiltz, J. (2006). The impact of behaviour problems on caregiver stress in young people with autism spectrum disorders. *Journal of Intellectual Disability Research, 50*(Pt 3), 172–183.

Marks, M. & Arkes, H. (2008). Patient and surrogate disagreement in end-of-life decisions: Can surrogates accurately predict patients' preferences? *Medical Decision Making, 28*(4), 524–531.

Moon, H., Townsend, A.L., Whitlatch, C.J., & Dilworth-Anderson, P. (2016). Quality of life for dementia caregiving dyads: Effects of incongruent perceptions of everyday care and values. *The Gerontologist.* doi: https://doi.org/10.1093/geront/gnw055

Nolan, M.R., Grant, G., & Ellis, N.C. (1990). Stress is in the eye of the beholder: Reconceptualizing the measurement of carer burden. *Journal of Advanced Nursing, 15*(5), 544–555.

O'Reilly, F., Finnan, F., Allwright, S., Smith, G.D., & Ben-Shlomo, Y. (1996). The effects of caring for a spouse with Parkinson's disease on social, psychological and physical well-being. *British Journal of General Practice, 46*(410), 507–512.

Pochard, F., Darmon, M., Fassier, T., Bollaert, P., Cheval, C., Coloigner, M., . . . Azoulay, E. (2005). Symptoms of anxiety and depression in family members of intensive care unit patients before discharge or death. A prospective multicenter study. *Journal of Critical Care, 20*(1), 90–96.

Schulz, R. & Sherwood, P.R. (2008). Physical and mental health effects of family caregiving. *American Journal of Nursing, 108*(9), 23–27.

Sharp, H. & Shega, J. (2009). Feeding tube placement in patients with advanced dementia: The beliefs and practice patterns of speech-language pathologists. *American Journal of Speech-Language Pathology, 18*(3), 222–230.

Stancin, T., Wade, S.L., Walz, N.C., Yeates, K.O., & Taylor, H.G. (2008). Traumatic brain injuries in early childhood: Initial impact on the family. *Journal of Developmental and Behavioral Pediatrics, 29*(4), 253-261.

Vitaliano, P.P., Zhang, J., & Scanlan, J.M. (2003). Is caregiving hazardous to one's physical health? A meta-analysis. *Psychological Bulletin, 129*(6), 946-972.

Whitlatch, C. (2008). Informal caregivers: Communication and decision making. *The American Journal of Nursing, 108*(9), 73-77.

5 Formal care contexts and professional carers

The empathetic clinician, and health beliefs, and the therapeutic relationship are concepts that most healthcare professionals think about constantly. There are many good texts regarding shared decision making and the empathetic listener. In this chapter, we discuss issues facing us as healthcare workers in the demanding environments we work in. We also discuss the issues facing the professional carers with whom we come into contact, who care for our patients on a daily basis. We use the term 'professional carers' to describe primarily paid carers who offer support to individual patients. This may include home care assistants, nurses or nursing auxiliaries. This group of people is responsible for daily care and for implementing the recommendations of other members of the healthcare team such as SLTs.

Caring professions

Compassion involves caring for other people, having sympathy for their condition and wanting to help them (Firth-Cozens & Cornwell, 2009; Parliamentary and Health Service Ombudsman, 2011). Compassionate care is a clear aim for healthcare organizations and is overtly articulated in some professional guidance. For other professions, the professional body directs their membership to relevant national documents. Examples of specific guidance include:

> "You put the interests of people using or needing nursing or midwifery services first. You make their care and safety your main concern and make sure that their dignity is preserved and their needs are recognised, assessed and responded to. You make sure that those receiving care are treated with respect, that their rights are upheld and that any discriminatory attitudes and behaviours towards those receiving care are challenged.

- 1 Treat people as individuals and uphold their dignity - to achieve this, you must:

    - 1.2 treat people with kindness, respect and compassion."

British Nursing: Prioritise people (Nursing & Midwifery Council, 2015)

"Physical therapist practice is guided by a set of seven core values: accountability, altruism, compassion/caring, excellence, integrity, professional duty, and social responsibility."

American Physical Therapy (APTA, 2010)

Complex relationships

When we begin an episode of care for a patient, the aim of the episode is for patients to receive the best evidence-based intervention, in a timely manner, with the outcome being what they want, within the bounds of what is medically feasible. In order to achieve optimal care, we must develop strong individualized relationships with our patients and their family or professional carers, so they have the confidence to discuss issues with us. Wagner (2006) defines a therapeutic relationship as the: "Mutually beneficial professional bond that exists between a healthcare professional and their patient" Wagner, 2006, p. 13).

This sounds simple but relationships are complex. The basis of a mutually beneficial relationship includes good communication, being honest and listening, trust and respect. We all know about the demands of a busy caseload, a hectic clinic, lots of community visits, pressure to make the maximum number of contacts in the minimum amount of time, good outcomes, productivity and value for money. And all that is without taking into consideration issues such as billable time, or number of sessions allocated for a given disability. Human relationships and their development are complex and often take time. So we begin to see that the creation and maintenance of the 'professional bond' is not as simple as it sounds.

Good quality care

Since the 1950s, the UK has had a nationalized health service. The aim of this health service is to:

"…improve our health and wellbeing, supporting us to keep mentally and physically well, to get better when we are ill and, when we cannot fully recover, to stay as well as we can to the end of our lives. It works at the limits of science – bringing the highest levels of human knowledge and skill to save lives and improve health. It touches our lives at times of basic human need, when care and compassion are what matter most"

Department of Health (2015, p. 2)

The constitution clearly states that care and compassion are central to good healthcare. Yet on a day-to-day basis, clinicians report barriers to offering a caring and compassionate service. Good leadership is essential for good quality care and to keep patients and their families at the centre of this care. The NHS Constitution describes the values that underpin health service delivery in the UK:

- Working together for patients – patients come first in everything we do

- Respect and dignity – we value every person whether patient, their families, or carers or staff

- Commitment to quality of care – we earn the trust placed in us by insisting on quality and striving to get the basics of quality of care – safety, effectiveness and patient experience – right every time

- Compassion – we ensure that compassion is central to the care we provide and respond with humanity and kindness to each person's pain, distress, anxiety or need

- Improving lives – we strive to improve health and wellbeing and people's experiences of the NHS

- Everyone counts – we maximise our resources for the whole of the community

Department of Health (2015, p. 5)

Even in countries that do not include healthcare or access to healthcare in their constitutions, such as the USA, we see that individual professions do (Swendiman, 2012). These values support the aspirations that the vast majority of us who came into healthcare have to make a difference to people's lives.

Challenges to caring

We live in difficult economic times and we have busy lives and many demands on our time. The Francis Report serves as a timely reminder about what can go wrong in healthcare when the wrong issues are prioritized (Francis, 2013). The vast majority of professionals go into their jobs with a desire to care for other people and they are dedicated, hardworking and professional staff. The Report also acknowledges that it is important and right that organizations are subject to financial and regulatory controls:

> "In introducing the first report, I said that it should be patients – not numbers – which counted. That remains my view. The demands for financial control, corporate governance, commissioning and regulatory systems are understandable and in many cases necessary. But it is not the system itself which will ensure that the patient is put first day in and day out. Any system should be capable of caring and delivering an acceptable level of care to each patient treated"
>
> (Francis, 2013)

The challenge is to remain motivated and caring professionals, delivering services with patients and families at the centre. We need to do this within the real and appropriate organizational and financial constraints that we work under.

The environments we work in are increasingly demanding and will continue to be so as patient complexity and longevity increase, financial constraints remain and the service and organizational contexts continue to change. This is the messy reality of working in healthcare. We could debate this throughout the chapter and never reach any useful conclusions. So we have chosen to acknowledge these challenges and set them on one side. We can then move forward with discussion about what makes good quality care and effective therapeutic relationships.

Working with professional carers

In the work that we do for our patients we are often reliant on working closely with professional carers. The underlying cause of the dysphagia, e.g., a stroke or cancer, often means that patients are reliant on support from professional care staff on a regular basis. Healthcare professionals rely on care staff to provide information during assessment, implement their recommendations on a daily basis, monitor the patient's presentation, and provide feedback (Crawford & Leslie, 2008; Davis & Copeland, 2005; Langmore et al., 1998; Rosenvinge & Starke, 2005; Wright, Cotter, & Hickson, 2008).

Estimates vary as to how closely professional carers follow recommendations for dysphagia. Recommendations are designed to ensure comfort and safety of individuals when eating and drinking. It is important that professional care staff follow recommendations closely because the evidence shows that where patients are dependent on other people for their oral intake, and more specifically need support for eating, they are more likely to be at risk for developing aspiration pneumonia, a serious consequence of dysphagia (Langmore et al., 1998). This risk may be exacerbated if recommendations are not followed closely. We must ensure that, while keeping our patient's wishes central, we also listen to care staff and to the challenges they face in order to work together to provide good quality care to our patients. It is important to remember that all patients should be monitored for intake, not just those with a dysphagia diagnosis label. Work with older people in the hospital setting has shown that those without a specific label often suffer from nutrition and hydration issues because their impairments are more subtle, for example, being too tired to complete a meal (Westergren, Unosson, Ohlsson, Lorefält, & Hallberg, 2002).

When professional care staff do not follow dysphagia recommendations, it is for a variety of reasons:

- Patient problems may be underestimated by care staff

- Care staff may not have adequate training knowledge and awareness

- There may not be enough staff to support each patient appropriately

- The staff may not have access to the correct equipment, utensils or texture modified food

- Lack of time.

(Colodny, 2001; Crawford, Leslie, & Drinnan, 2007; Rosenvinge & Starke, 2005).

Care staff often do not follow recommendations because they are too much 'hassle' (Colodny, 2001). Care staff tend to follow recommendations if they believe that the patient's problem is of genuine concern, and if they have belief in the efficacy of the treatment. Equally concerning for staff is when a patient prefers to continue oral eating despite professional recommendations. In this case the clinical professional responsible may find that their role is to advocate for the patient and to provide education and support to the care staff (Serradura-Russell, 1992). Staff's perception of what feeding is about may also affect action such as whether it is about socialising or biomechanical nutrition (Pelletier, 2005). This has implications for ensuring adequate knowledge and training for care staff. These studies suggest that in order to improve the ability of professional carers to follow our recommendations SLTs need to engage in the following activities:

- Provide training to care staff so that they understand what dysphagia is, why implementing recommendations is important, and what they need to do for their individual patients specifically

- Collaborate on writing guidelines, to give care staff an understanding and some ownership over the guidelines, and listen to their perspective

- Encourage access to good support and supervision from within their organizations, and initiatives such as 'dysphagia link nurse' schemes may help

(Rosenvinge & Starke, 2005)

- Provide ongoing support ourselves so that care staff have a chance to review our recommendations and their responsibilities, to ask questions and to update their knowledge.

These challenges are faced by care staff at the micro level: they are related to the individual patient, the individual carer, the specific ward or kitchen. But these challenges link to, and are often exacerbated by, challenges at a more macro level. These issues have been highlighted by the recent literature about compassion.

Compassion and therapeutic relationships

If we consider the challenges to caring that were presented earlier in this chapter we must acknowledge that most staff come to work to do a good job, and are aiming to be compassionate and caring, but conditions sometimes make it difficult for them:

> "...it was not because nurses had lost their compassion... changes in the NHS and the demands put on nurses distracted them from being compassionate"
>
> (Black, 2008, p. 10)

The context that professional carers now work in is often reported to prevent compassionate care being possible. The context is reported as:

> "too complex, fast paced and demanding"
>
> (Dewar & Christley, 2013, p. 48)

> "critical focus on pathways, tasks and documentation... ever-increasing demand on acute care systems and staff shortages"
>
> (Youngson, 2011, p. 7)

> "external agendas must be met, quality...boxes demand attention to ensure payment...whether or not these are evidence based or benefit the individual patient concerned... costs require rationing"
>
> (Knight, 2011, p. 51).

Despite a wish to care and be compassionate, it remains challenging for professional carers. We have to balance these challenges with drivers in healthcare internationally, that instruct us and our professional care colleagues to focus on providing compassionate care against a backdrop of difficult working environments and demands (Firth-Cozens & Cornwell, 2009; Najjar, Davis, Beck-Coon, & Carney Doebbeling, 2009).

Youngson points out how traditional medical models encourage both detachment from patients and the belief that to stay detached and remote from patients prevents health practitioners from become burnt out (Youngson, 2011). Youngson counters this argument, as he feels that engaging with patients, being compassionate and enjoying a human relationship may prevent professional care staff from becoming fatigued from the effort of caring. This is a fine balance to develop in a novice clinician and points to the need for good supervision, especially in the period after qualification and ideally as a career-long activity. In countries or facilities where productivity drives healthcare we need to be particularly mindful of our less experienced colleagues and what they take home or off the clock to get their jobs done.

The literature concerned with the concept of compassion provides some concrete advice about how to increase compassion in the workplace, at an operational level, i.e., what professional carers do 'on the floor', and at a strategic level, i.e., how managers and leaders think about and embed compassion throughout their organizations. This advice sits neatly with the literature that considers therapeutic relationships. We need to consider compassion for our patients, and compassion for the care staff we work with, who are often working in difficult circumstances. We also need to encourage compassion in the approach of the care staff towards our patients. We said at the start that relationships are complex. In order for our patients to receive the support that they need, we need to be thinking about relationships on many levels.

On an individual level, we must encourage care staff to reflect on their own behaviours to ensure compassionate care because patients report that they need to feel the 'human' aspect of care. Evidence going back to the 1950s, but summarized by Greenhalgh and Heath (2010), indicates that patients need to feel:

> "...friendship, respect, commitment, affirmation, recognition, responsiveness, positive regard, empathy, trust, receptivity, alignment between the doctor's agenda and that of the patient's life world"
>
> (Greenhalgh & Heath, 2010, p. 4)

Many of the components listed above are common to any caring human relationship. Within healthcare the challenge now is to 'humanize healthcare' (de Zulueta, 2013, p. 89). We can draw together a list of behaviours from the literature that encapsulate compassionate behaviour, and allow care staff to develop more therapeutic relationships with patients (de Zulueta, 2013 ; O'Brien, 2006; Pullen & Mathias, 2010; Youngson, 2011). As care staff ourselves, we need to take time to reflect on our own behaviours and ensure that we are engaging in positive relationships with our patients and our care staff colleagues. These behaviours focus on developing and using good communication skills at every level:

- Start at the very beginning by introducing yourself and using the name of the person to whom you are talking

- Actively listen and stop talking, maintain appropriate eye contact and display empathy for what you are being told

- Prioritize the need to spend time with people to listen and communicate

- Use the information you are given to offer appropriate support, learn and develop – learn particularly from patient stories

- Engage in regular communication with colleagues

- Make time to reflect on your practice, and create an environment where open and honest reflection, and sharing concerns about your own performance is acceptable and regular supervision is encouraged.

(Granger, 2014; Kahn, 2008)

Most importantly, for this to take place the organization has to adopt "compassion as a core value" (Youngson, 2011, p. 7). This allows staff to embrace these compassionate values with support and without fear of recrimination.

The NHS in the UK has produced its *Vision and Strategy for Nurses, Midwives and Care Staff*, which aims to embed good communication skills in the practice of all staff, in a 'Culture of Compassionate Care' underpinned by the 6 Cs – care, compassion, competence, communication, courage, commitment. This is an update on the 6 Cs first introduced by Emanuel and Dubler in 1995, which demonstrates the requirement to continually strive to ensure we demonstrate these behaviours in our practice, and review and reflect on the way we interact with patients and care staff, and the way care staff interact with patients on our behalf (Emanuel & Dubler, 1995).

So what does this mean for dysphagia?

Nan lives in a care home. At the moment, the care home she lives in is understaffed and the staff who are still working there are working long hours and are tired. They have to complete their daily duties which involve housework as well as offering direct support to the patients who live in the house. They also have paperwork to fill in at key points during the day. The staff are unhappy and stressed. Nan had a choking episode about two weeks ago. She is meant to have 1:1 support during mealtimes but on the day in question an inexperienced member of staff was on duty, serving the food for the six residents in the home as well as keeping an eye on the four who need supervision and support at mealtimes.

Nan's eating and drinking recommendations, which have been agreed using the legal framework of best interests decision making, state that she should have a soft, moist, well chopped diet. The new member of staff had thought that a warm sausage roll cut up into squares met this criterion. Nan stopped breathing and required abdominal thrusts to dislodge the piece of sausage role. The member of staff was only aware there was a problem when other residents alerted her to the fact Nan was not well. Following the event there was an internal investigation and the senior carer has now placed Nan on a fully liquidized diet. The new member of staff has been taken off all duties that involve direct care for any of the residents. Nan is now extremely unhappy and distressed and indicates that she want to eat like the other residents. She is asking for her favourite foods: fish pie and spaghetti bolognese. The senior member of staff says that she knows that Nan wants to go back to the diet she had previously and that she hates the liquidized diet. Ten years ago, the senior member of staff witnessed someone choking to death, and says that while Nan hates the diet she's on surely this is better than the risk of choking again. She says she also never wants to go through the investigation process again, and that the paperwork involved was dreadful.

On review of this case it is possible that if the recommendations for Nan had been followed it would be unlikely that she would have choked. The change to a pureed diet has been done to reduce fear and pressure in the already stressed staff group. Due to the level of stress in the staff home, it is possible the staff will find it difficult to be compassionate, caring and person-centred with Nan. Fear in relation to the previous choking episode may also be significant. It is important to really listen to staff groups about the pressures they are under, the concerns they have, and to work together to help understand the patient's difficulties and develop person-centred care plans. During such dialogue, people may feel listened to and less scared so compromise is more likely.

Once this understanding is reached it may be appropriate in a case like Nan's to work closely with the staff group and offer formal training and ongoing support that compromise and show understanding of the facility pressures. As staff feel more confident it then may be possible to arrive at a more person-centred set of recommendations for Nan.

Henry has been admitted to hospital with a serious chest infection. During his stay in hospital his mother reports that she overheard the nurses talking with the doctor responsible for his care. The doctor was explaining to the nurses that his swallowing problems have caused his chest infection. The doctor says that it is clear that, because of the nature of his swallowing problems, eating and drinking will not be a pleasure for him, that he will have no quality of life and that a feeding tube will be the best thing for him. Henry's mother is very upset about this because she feels that the doctor is not viewing Henry as an individual and is making assumptions about Henry's condition, what he takes pleasure from, and his quality of life.

Compassionate care requires putting the patient at the centres of intervention and not making assumptions about what a patient might want based on our own values and beliefs. This can be difficult when working in envirnmentsenvironments that are busy and provide us with little opportunity to get to know our patients. Professional carers act in a proxy capacity on our behalf, implementing recommendations for our patients. Difficult working environments can get in the way of providing person-centred compassionate care. Relationships between healthcare professionals, patients and families are complex and should be therapeutic. This requires healthcare professionals to work together with families and patients, listen to the views of all those involved, and collaborate to implement the right treatment plans for individuals.

References

APTA. (2010). Code of Ethics for the Physical Therapist. Retrieved 26 May 2016, from http://www.apta.org/uploadedFiles/APTAorg/About_Us/Policies/Ethics/CodeofEthics.pdf

Black, S. (2008). The power of compassion. *Nursing Standard, 23*(7), 70-71.

Colodny, N. (2001). Construction and validation of the mealtime and dysphagia questionnaire: An instrument designed to assess nursing staff reasons for noncompliance with SLP dysphagia and feeding recommendations. *Dysphagia, 16*(4), 263-271.

Crawford, H. & Leslie, P. (2008). Pushing interdisciplinary boundaries. *Bulletin, Jan,* 20-21.

Crawford, H., Leslie, P., & Drinnan, M. (2007). Compliance with dysphagia recommendations by carers of adults with intellectual impairment. *Dysphagia, 22*(4), 326-334.

Davis, L. & Copeland, K. (2005). Effectiveness of computer-based dysphagia training for direct patient care staff. *Dysphagia, 20*(2), 141-148.

de Zulueta, P. (2013). Compassion in healthcare. *Clinical Ethics, 8*(4), 87-90.

Department of Health. (2015, 27 July). The NHS Constititution. Retrieved 22 May 2016, from https://www.gov.uk/government/uploads/system/uploads/attachment_data/file/480482/NHS_Constitution_WEB.pdf

Dewar, B. & Christley, Y. (2013). A critical analysis of compassion in practice. *Nursing Standard, 28*(10), 46-50.

Emanuel, E. J. & Dubler, N.N. (1995). Preserving the physician-patient relationship in the era of managed care. *JAMA, 273*(4), 323-329.

Firth-Cozens, J. & Cornwell, J. (2009). The point of care: Enabling compassionate care in acute hospital settings. London: The King's Fund.

Francis, R. (2013). *Report of the Mid Staffordshire NHS Foundation Trust Public Inquiry: Executive Summary.* (9780102981476). London: Her Majesty's Stationery Office. Retrieved from http://webarchive.nationalarchives.gov.uk/20150407084003/http://www.midstaffspublicinquiry.com/sites/default/files/report/Executive%20summary.pdf

Granger, K. (2014). Hello My Name Is... Retrieved 30 December 2015, from http://hellomynameis.org.uk/

Greenhalgh, T. & Heath, I. (2010). Measuring quality in the therapeutic relationship. In T.K.S. Fund (Ed.), *An Inquiry into the Quality of General Practice in England.* London: The King's Fund.

Kahn, M. (2008). Etiquette-based medicine. *New England Journal of Medicine, 358*(19), 1988-1989.

Knight, R. (2011). The doctor, the patient and compassion. *Journal of Holistic Healthcare, 8*(3), 50-53.

Langmore, S.E., Terpenning, M.S., Schork, A., Chen, Y., Murray, J.T., Lopatin, D., & Loesche, W.J. (1998). Predictors of aspiration pneumonia: How important is dysphagia? *Dysphagia, 13*(2), 69-81.

Najjar, N., Davis, L.W., Beck-Coon, K., & Carney Doebbeling, C. (2009). Compassion fatigue: A review of the research to date and relevance to cancer-care providers. *Journal of Health Psychology, 14*(2), 267-277.

Nursing & Midwifery Council. (2015). The Code: Professional standards of practice and behaviour for nurses and midwives. Retrieved 26 May 2016, from https://www.nmc. org.uk/standards/code/read-the-code-online/

O'Brien, P. J. (2006). Creating compassion and connection in the work place. *Journal of Systemic Therapies, 25*(1), 16-36.

Parliamentary and Health Service Ombudsman. (2011). Care and compassion? Report of the Health Service Ombudsman on ten investigations into NHS care of older people, from http://www.ombudsman.org.uk/__data/assets/pdf_file/0016/7216/Care-and-Compassion-PHSO-0114web.pdf

Pelletier, C.A. (2005). Feeding beliefs of certified nurse assistants in the nursing home: A factor influencing practice. *Journal of Gerontological Nursing, 31*(7), 5-10.

Pullen, R.L. & Mathias, T. (2010). Fostering therapeutic nurse-patient relationships. *Nursing Made Incredibly Easy!, May/June*, 4.

Rosenvinge, S.K. & Starke, I.D. (2005). Improving care for patients with dysphagia. *Age & Ageing, 34*(6), 587-593.

Serradura-Russell, A. (1992). Ethical dilemmas in dysphagia management and the right to a natural death. *Dysphagia, 7*(2), 102-105.

Swendiman, K.S. (2012). Health care: Constitutional rights and legislative powers. *CRS Report for Congress.* Retrieved 26 May 2016, from https://www.fas.org/sgp/crs/misc/R40846.pdf

Wagner, M. (2006). *Exploring the Therapeutic Relationship: Practical Insights for Today's Clinician.* Sandy, UT: Aardvark Global Publishing.

Westergren, A., Unosson, M., Ohlsson, O., Lorefält, B., & Hallberg, I. (2002). Eating difficulties, assisted eating and nutritional status in elderly (>=65 years) patients in hospital rehabilitation. *International Journal of Nursing Studies, 39*(3), 341-351.

Wright, L., Cotter, D., & Hickson, M. (2008). The effectiveness of targeted feeding assistance to improve the nutritional intake of elderly dysphagic patients in hospital. *Journal of Human Nutrition & Dietetics, 21*(6), 555-562; quiz 564-555.

Youngson, R. (2011). Compassion in healthcare. *Journal of Holistic Healthcare, 8*(3), 6-9.

6 Frameworks

We have used the term 'framework' as opposed to guidelines or protocols because frameworks are not prescriptive instructions on how one arrives at a good decision. Frameworks are more than topic areas to be considered and then infused into our general thinking. A framework suggests structure and support. Legally and professionally we will stand on surer ground if we can show a systematic approach to our work rather than citing 'intuition' or 'experience'. Whilst experience is definitely a requirement for a clinician to develop good working practice it is not enough to defend decisions. Empathy for our patients and family carers is equally important but again, not defensible on its own.

Values, morals and ethics

The terms 'values', 'morals' and 'ethics' are used interchangeably and without much thought by most of us. If we pause to reflect on their exact meanings things become cloudy. Definitions will vary depending on the source we consult. We map the three terms broadly to the definitions given by ChangingMinds. org (Straker, 2016). It is important to separate 'values', 'morals' and 'ethics' as a way of parsing out what might be influencing different parties that are trying to come to a decision on something. Because an individual's view of what is 'right' or 'wrong' is based on his/her personal value system and then aligned with a cultural map (morals) we can find it very difficult to appreciate that another person's way of thinking is equally 'right' albeit different to our own.

Values

> "Values are the rules by which we make decisions about right and wrong, should and shouldn't, good and bad. They also tell us which are more or less important, which is useful when we have to trade off meeting one value over another."
>
> (Straker, 2016)

Values are highly personal: we develop them over time and they are influenced by our social groups. Thus we get some values from our family, some from friends, and some from cultural groups that are important to us. This might include an ethnic culture such as being Japanese or a social culture such as being a member of a political party. Professions and work settings also have a 'culture' if you consider how people think in an acute hospital compared to those working in community residential homes, for example.

The idea of trading or ranking values comes up every day for us. Let us say that two of my values are loyalty to friends and fidelity in relationships. I have a friend called Syd that I have known since I was five years of age. She is in a committed relationship and I am friends with her partner Chris. One day I find out that my childhood friend is having an affair. Chris - my friend also – confides in me a worry that Syd is seeing someone else and wonders what to do. So now I have to rank my thoughts on loyalty against those on fidelity. Whatever I do I will rank one value over another.

Morals

"Morals have a greater social element to values and tend to have a very broad acceptance. Morals are far more about good and bad than other values. We thus judge others more strongly on morals than values."

(Straker, 2016)

Morals are society's value system if you like. This is where we can see major clashes as the society we live and work in becomes more multicultural. We are often not conscious of where our feelings come from about what is culturally acceptable - we just feel that Mr Smith is being 'awkward' in his reluctance to discuss some aspect of his clinical care. Once we start discussing matters it turns out that he was brought up to not question his elders, or revered members of the community. In real life this means that Mr Smith does not want to 'discuss' things because he feels it is disrespectful.

As an individual we might find ourselves in conflict internally. I might live in a society where healthcare is more or less available depending on social factors such as wealth or education. And yet where I was trained - my professional 'culture' – instilled a sense of access to my care for all. So my employment will not support my professionally autonomous decision to treat Mr Lee for more weeks of therapy.

Ethics

> "Ethics tend to be codified into a formal system or set of rules which are explicitly adopted by a group of people. Thus you have medical ethics. Ethics are thus internally defined and adopted, whilst morals tend to be externally imposed on other people. If you accuse someone of being unethical, it is equivalent of calling them unprofessional and may well be taken as a significant insult and perceived more personally than if you called them immoral (which of course they may also not like)."
>
> (Straker, 2016)

We will discuss *Medical Ethics* shortly but under this concept of ethics are our Professional Codes (The Royal College of Speech and Language Therapists, 2006), Health & Care Professions Council in the UK (Health & Care Professions Council, 2016), or the American Speech-Language Hearing Association in the USA (American Speech-Language-Hearing Association, 2016). A professional code of ethics is a set of rules that members of that body must follow: if you want to be in our gang these are the *dos* and *do nots*.

When we find ourselves in a decision making process where things are becoming more difficult or communication has broken down it is useful to step back and ask ourselves why? Is the sticking point really a clash of professional position, e.g., the physician is pushing eating because she is the one in charge and the SLT is pushing nil orally because swallow advice is *his turf*, or is this really a reflection of their different moral backgrounds (perhaps deeply religious)? When the mother of our patient is 'combative' and 'unreasonable', is it that she ranks her role as *nurturing person who feeds* higher than her value of *deferring to professionals* (which she may also hold but at some point she may have to rank one above the other).

Evidence based practice

Evidence based practice is a term that all in healthcare are familiar with. But not all can define it or apply it to clinical situations even several decades after it started to appear in practice guidelines. In the 1990s we started to see publications defining *evidence based medicine*. Typically there was reference to the deliberate and judicious use of *best evidence* by someone with clinical expertise to support decision making in the care of a patient. *Best* evidence was taken to be *external* to the clinician and generally the product of robust research. Such a framework sounds sensible. We presume that good clinicians have expertise due to their experience of working with certain conditions and situations (*internal evidence*). These clinicians will maintain their competence by using scientific literature (*external evidence*) to support their own thoughts. Equipped with such internal and external evidence the expert will suggest approaches to an illness or a situation and the patient's values and preferences will be incorporated.

In the early days the patient perspective was rarely mentioned. We would encourage people to read the seminal article by Sackett and his colleagues from 1996, "Evidence based medicine: what it is and isn't" (Sackett, Rosenberg, Gray, Haynes, & Richardson, 1996). Although this part is not often quoted Sackett et al were very clear on what it means to be a 'clinical expert':

> "Increased expertise is reflected in many ways, but especially in more effective and efficient diagnosis and in the **more thoughtful identification and compassionate use of individual patients' predicaments, rights, and preferences** in making clinical decisions about their care."

> (Sackett et al., 1996), p. 71, our emphasis)

From early on the patient perspective was a fundamental component of evidence based medicine. How did this component get quietly forgotten for so long? Perhaps because of the "distortion of the evidence based brand" by parties with interests other than those of the patient or clinician, argues Trisha Greenhalgh and colleagues in a recent BMJ publication (Greenhalgh, Howick, & Maskrey, 2014, p.1).

Evidence based medicine is often represented as in Figure 1, with the ideal practice occurring at the centre supported by the three tenets.

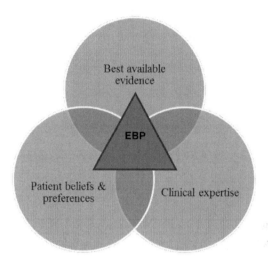

Figure 1 Traditional evidence based medicine (practice)

The Cochrane Collaboration takes this a step further and looks at evidence based clinical practice which they define as:

> "an approach to decision-making in which the clinician uses the best evidence available, in consultation with the patient, to decide upon the option which suits that patient best"

> (The Cochrane Collaboration, 2014)

Here the shift is to consult the patient but still it requires interpretation as the clinician decides on the best fit for the patient. What about patient autonomy – we will address this in the section on Medical Principles. Is it fair to ask the patient to make such weighty judgements? After all, they came to us because we are 'experts'. We propose that the traditional picture of evidence based practice should be modified as in Figure 2.

Conscious use of the word *informed* reminds us firstly that clinicians are not experts because they have been working for many years, or they (and others) consider them to be 'eminent'. An informed expert regularly tempers and expands their knowledge by attending the lectures of other experts, by listening to stakeholders in the same area of interest, which for us is the patient and family, other healthcare workers, the kitchen staff, and others. We must

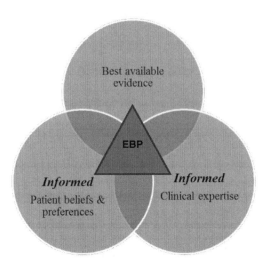

Figure 2 Evidence based practice update

triangulate across sources and we have a duty to reflect on our practice (Katz, 2002). Sackett et al. used the word 'thoughtful' in the quote above which to us equates to the reflective practice that is part of our professional identity.

Medical principles

In bioethics the *Principles* approach relies on considering an issue with respect to a set of principles. These principles are said to be "culturally neutral" (Gillon, 1994, p.184) but we must accept that they were founded in a Western philosophical approach to personhood and relevant to the medical model. Bioethicists and philosophers argue about the appropriateness and neutrality of this model and that debate is beyond the focus of our book. We mention this only to alert people to the perspective that, for example, autonomy as an *individual's* right is a Western concept and that medical and legal frameworks are founded on this for healthcare decisions is not a universal view. Many Eastern cultures consider autonomy to be a social group responsibility. In Eastern cultures major decisions on healthcare, life and death, even for western -trained physicians who are ill, may be defaulted to the family (Kleinman, 1988).

Medical ethical principles, as they are now known, are based on the work by Tom Beauchamp and James Childress who identified a set of moral duties that clinicians should align their work with:

- To respect and enable autonomy

- To act beneficently

- To act nonmaleficently

- To ensure justice.

(Beauchamp & Childress, 2013)

We find this framework useful because it makes us consider several aspects to an issue. We may well be familiar with the words in a colloquial sense but putting a patient at the centre of the principles will help us to gain some clarity and acknowledge the difficult grey areas.

We also need to consider when and/or how to apply the principles. This has been concisely explained in a paper by Gillon who outlined the four principles and then took us a step further and showed us how to consider the scope of our duty (Gillon, 1994). Our *Scope* is our patient(s) and we are to act with beneficence towards them. He does touch upon the grey area of scope and autonomy for those who are very young or with diminished cognitive abilities. Wisely he counsels us that we need to think of the specific decision to be made by the individual rather than presuming autonomy or not based on age or intelligence. This harks back to the idea of a person having capacity for a specific decision at a specific time (see Chapter 3).

Autonomy

Autonomy is often thought of as the number one principle: I must respect this person (my patient) purely because they are another human being. They have the right to decide what is done to them, or *not* done to them. We must as clinical professionals ensure that we are enabling autonomy which is not simply a matter of letting patients pick any intervention they wish. Similarly, we must appreciate that patients may not know all of their options and they *do not know which questions to ask* in order to find out about those options. It is part of our duty of care to enable patients to ask the right questions so that they may have the information that they need for their particular scenario.

In the late 20th century two things combined to influence patient choice. One was the increasing familiarity with the concept of patient 'autonomy'. The second was the move to view healthcare in a similar way to other business transactions. Clinicians felt under increasing pressure to agree to anything the patient (or family) wanted in order to demonstrate that they were respecting 'patient autonomy'. As more clinicians gave in to patient demands irrespective of the appropriateness it became the normal standard of care. If a patient was not offered or refused a particular intervention they might react badly – why were they being *deprived of their right*? Autonomy is not supported when we simply agree to a patient's request for something medically futile or even irrelevant. Clinicians need to make certain that patients are well-informed about costs and benefits of different options – only this supports patients in making autonomous decisions.

Beneficence

Beneficence is the act of doing good and removing harm. Clinicians would be horrified to think that they were not doing good or not removing harm. To maintain clinical competence relating to the interventions (assessment or therapy) that I might propose, I must have a good educational foundation and continually update my knowledge. We must step back and reflect on *good for whom*? What is the net good of our approach once we have weighed its costs against its benefits? For most interventions there are no absolutes; instead they tend to result in 'an increased risk of this' or 'less chance of that'. For some patients it may be that they can have some oral intake despite clinical findings indicating problems because the personal and social wellbeing that is derived outweighs the *possible* increase in aspiration. There has been recent debate about policies on 'risk feeding' but we caution against the use of this term given that all eating and drinking carries risk (choking, food poisoning) and the term infers a weighting towards oral feeding being the *bad* thing.

Nonmaleficence

The act of causing harm to a patient is surely an anathema to any clinician. But *harm* must be considered in the broad sense: loss of activity due to restrictive practice, isolation due to embarrassment of the techniques one has been advised to use to lessen the alleged risk with swallowing, or treating a patient whom we are not competent to deal with. The evidence supporting the use of altered consistency of food/drink is minimal. We do have evidence that people on thickened liquids drink less and the same with altered consistency food (Robbins et al., 2008; Wright, Cotter, Hickson, & Frost, 2005). We would argue that putting someone on a restrictive diet introduces a known cost to them, which may be viewed as deliberately increasing a patient's risk for harm.

Justice

To deliver just healthcare we need to supply what people *need* in a *fair* way. How do we work out what people *need*? This requires the process of dialogue, that is a back and forth discussion with the stakeholders involved. Establishing what people need cannot be done by simply advising what we think is best based on our expertise. Being fair requires us to think beyond the one person in front of us: what resources do we have across the full caseload, what might be the effect on the whole family, what evidence is there that our proposed intervention is effective in this population group and/or this specific type of case?

Broader structures: The Seedhouse Grid

In thinking of healthcare intervention, effects and resources in a broader fashion it is useful to have a framework that acknowledges this and the Ethical Grid is one such structure (Seedhouse, 2009). There are four layers to the Grid (see Figure 3):

- Core concepts, e.g., create and respect autonomy, respect persons equally, serve needs first

- Moral duties and motives, e.g., minimize harm (nonmaleficence), do the most good (beneficence), tell the truth (veracity), keep promise (fidelity)s

- Outcomes and priorities, e.g., most beneficial outcome for the patient, most beneficial outcome for a particular group, most beneficial outcome for society, most beneficial outcome for oneself

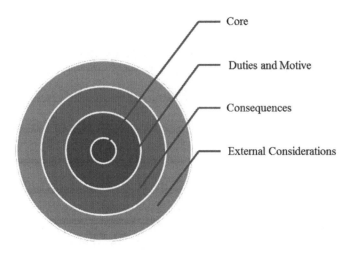

Figure 3 Ethical Grid Approach (Seedhouse, 2009)

- Practicalities, e.g., available resources, codes of practice, the law, wishes of others, the degree of certainty of the evidence on which the action is taken.

We strongly encourage you to read *Ethics: The Heart of Healthcare* to gain an appreciation of the background to this work and for its good case examples (Seedhouse, 2009). The idea behind this grid is that we are forced to look broadly at aspects relative to a healthcare decision. This covers a range of issues from the most central tenets of health care to what might be legal or available in our particular setting. Before overriding our moral obligations as health care professionals we must think carefully. Recommending a theoretically superior intervention but not considering the practicalities of availability or impact on, say, the family is not a good outcome for a decision making process.

Best interests decision making

We have discussed the legal framework around capacity in chapter 3. If a patient is able to make decisions about their health for themselves, then following the frameworks discussed we can support patients to go ahead with the treatment that suits them. When we are sure that an individual cannot make their own decisions about an assessment or intervention we need to work with family and professional carers to help make decisions about which treatment options are in the best interests of the patient. In situations where a patient's capacity will return we can defer some decisions but may have to go ahead with surrogacy if urgent action is needed. It is important to consult all relevant parties about what they feel is the best for the patient based on their knowledge and relationship with the patient. There is no specific definition of *best interests,* rather a checklist of things that must be considered when making a decision on behalf of another (Office of the Public Guardian, 2005). This includes making sure that the patient's capacity will not return to a point where they could make their own decision, taking into account any previous beliefs or wishes of the patient, and ensuring that any decisions are not made on the basis of age, appearance, condition or behaviour.

There are also frameworks available to help protect vulnerable adults which clinicians may need to consult if they have concerns that their patient is at risk of abuse. These frameworks may vary in name or description dependent on the host country, but they tend to use terms such as 'safeguarding adults' or 'adult protection'. Abuse can come in many forms – financial, physical, emotional, sexual and neglect, and a vulnerable adult may suffer abuse from anyone they come into contact with. The patients we work with often fall into a group of adults who are vulnerable to abuse, in that they may have reduced communicative or cognitive ability, physical disabilities, reduced awareness, limited support, or they may be frail or elderly. Practitioners should seek out support from the appropriate agencies in their host country should they suspect a patient is at risk of or experiencing abuse.

How is this relevant to decisions in dysphagia?

Following her stroke, Geethu-Joseph and her family have received advice from the health team that recommends that she should have a well mashed diet, and drink her fluids from a double handled spouted cup. Geethu-Joseph and her family are very unhappy with these recommendations and this is causing conflict within the family and between the family and the health team.

Resolving the conflict within the family and between the family and the health team may be challenging. Considering values, morals and ethics may help us view these challenges from different perspectives. Health professionals often make recommendations based on their values, morals and ethics both as health professionals and as individual human beings. Values will include what they rank as important, and may involve values in relation to keeping Geethu-Joseph as physically well as possible and the medial ethics they see as their professional responsibility to follow. As far as Geethu-Joseph and her family are concerned, the values, morals and ethics may differ. Untangling and articulating these will be the key to getting the intervention right for Geethu-Joseph and her family and resolving conflict within all the relationships. Personal values will affect how a person will calculate 'net good'.

Practitioners should be encouraged to think about the relative certainty of the costs they fear, such as choking or aspirating, which are different and allow different diets. Consider what other approaches could be used, for example establishing which foods in the family's usual diet fit the soft ideal but are normally prepared that way rather than mashing all foods which may appear infantile. What does the double handed cup help with, and could that need be approached in a different way that suits all stakeholders goals.

Henry has been re-referred to the health team because his physical condition is deteriorating. He is losing weight and the care staff at his day facility are concerned that he is coughing increasingly on all food and fluid and has had several chest infections in the last six weeks. On full assessment of his condition from a range of health professionals the health team feel that he would benefit from enteral support for the majority of his nutrition and hydration. Henry's cognitive difficulties have been assessed and indicate they are such that he is not able to understand the information or decision. Henry's parents are adamant that he enjoys his food and that at home he has no difficulties. They are opposed to any suggestion of enteral feeding.

Using the evidence based practice framework can help health teams, patients and families structure discussions and address all important aspects of the decision to be made. The evidence based practice framework supports us to consider the best available evidence that is relevant to the decision to be made, so we can search out good quality literature to help us in our clinical discussions. We should also factor in our own clinical experience and that of the rest of the health team. The practitioner should reflect on similar cases and their outcomes with the team and supervisor. The wishes of the patient and family should be considered and given equal amount of weight as the evidence and experience components.

Using a framework helps us look at all aspects of the decision in a balanced way and to uncover our blindspots. It can also help patients and families understand the factors the team may be considering in coming to recommendations. To continue to develop as professionals we should discuss cases in clinical supervision so that all aspects of the case management can be considered. Clinical supervision helps us think through and reflect on cases, and to explore a range of options. We can then present the options for discussion with the patient. Clinical supervision is the cornerstone of robust, good quality intervention and should be an essential part of our clinical practice. Ultimately Henry's safety may have to be put above that of his family's preferences but this should only happen after full discussion, over a period of time and when the family has been encouraged to voice all of their concerns *and* have been listened to.

References

American Speech-Language-Hearing Association. (1 March, 2016). Code of Ethics. Retrieved 10 March 2016, from http://www.asha.org/Code-of-Ethics/

Beauchamp, T.L., & Childress, J.F. (2013). *Principles of Biomedical Ethics* (7th ed.). New York: Oxford University Press.

Gillon, R. (1994). Medical ethics: Four principles plus attention to scope. *BMJ, 309*(6948), 184.

Greenhalgh, T., Howick, J., & Maskrey, N. (2014). Evidence based medicine: a movement in crisis? *BMJ, 348*, g3725.

Health & Care Professions Council. (2016). *Your duties as a registrant: Standards of conduct, performance and ethics.* (20120801POLPUB/SCPE (updated January 2016)). London: Health & Care Professions Council. Retrieved from http://www.hcpc-uk.org/assets/do cuments/10004EDFStandardsofconduct,performanceandethics.pdf

Katz, J. (2002). *The Silent World of Doctor and Patient.* Baltimore: Johns Hopkins University Press.

Kleinman, A. (1988). Illness unto death. *The Illness Narratives* (Chapter 9, pp. 146-157). New York: Basic Books.

Office of the Public Guardian. (2005, 22 October 2014). Mental Capacity Act. Retrieved 26 May, 2016, from https://www.justice.gov.uk/protecting-the-vulnerable/mental-capacity-act

Robbins, J., Gensler, G., Hind, J., Logemann, J.A., Lindblad, A.S., Brandt, D., . . . Miller Gardner, P.J. (2008). Comparison of 2 interventions for liquid aspiration on pneumonia incidence: A randomized trial. *Annals of Internal Medicine, 148*(7), 509–518.

Sackett, D.L., Rosenberg, W.M., Gray, J.A., Haynes, R.B., & Richardson, W.S. (1996). Evidence based medicine: What it is and what it isn't. *BMJ, 312*(7023), 71–72.

Seedhouse, D. (2009). *Ethics: The Heart of Healthcare* (Third ed.). Chichester: John Wiley & Sons.

Straker, D. (2016). Values, morals, ethics. Retrieved 26 May 2016, from http://www.changingminds.org/explanations/values/values_morals_ethics.htm

The Cochrane Collaboration. (26 May 2014). Evidence-based health care and systematic reviews. Retrieved 14 June, from http://www.cochrane.org/about-us/evidence-based-health-care#REF1

The Royal College of Speech and Language Therapists. (2006). *Communicating Quality 3: RCSLT's Guidance on Best Practice in Service Organisation and Provision*. London: The Royal College of Speech and Language Therapists.

Wright, L., Cotter, D., Hickson, M., & Frost, G. (2005). Comparison of energy and protein intakes of older people consuming a texture modified diet with a normal hospital diet. *Journal of Hum Nutrition and Diet, 18*(3), 213–219.

7 Summary

Bioethics and decisions in dysphagia

Let us hark back to where we started with this concept: "bioethicists seek to figure out what people should do" (National Institutes for Health, 2009). We propose that thinking about frameworks that we are more familiar with, such as evidence-based practice, in conjunction with a bioethical approach helps us to make more sense of resources with which we are familiar. Most healthcare professionals are swimming in guidelines and protocols, care pathways and regulations, and yet decision making has not got easier. Taking a step back helps us to think more broadly and in closer alignment with other professionals. We become familiar with some common language of the medical and legal worlds. More importantly, this bigger picture view will help us to contribute to improved and robust decision making with our patients. Our rationale for a given action is more defensible, be it regarding a new treatment approach or supporting a patient to optimize their situation despite refusing our ideal recommendations.

The central character

Big picture approaches can be successfully combined with the life and healthcare of an individual. The patient is the person living with and experiencing the illness that we as a clinician can only diagnose as a disease. Thus, for any decision to be defensible it must start with the patient. We must understand the context that our patient is situated in, which may involve family or professional carers, and their needs and restrictions require consideration.

Know thyself

The Ancient Greek maxim 'know thyself' was inscribed in the Temple of Apollo at Delphi in the 2nd century AD according to a geographer of the time, Pausanias (Pretzler, 2007). Interpretations of what this means vary from judging yourself before you judge others, to ignoring the multitudes' perceptions of you. How does it apply to our discussions? We have encouraged you to look outwards at other people, other disciplines, and other frameworks in order to support working with patients and families. Some evaluation of our work in-house should also be undertaken. A significant contribution to poor decision making lies at our own door.

We need to carefully consider how and what we advise on, and how we communicate our ideas. Clinical competency and knowledge of our Scope of Practice is taught from early in our training. We spend far less time addressing how we communicate between speech and language therapists regarding our findings, and how others might (mis)interpret our words. For example, if a patient is based in the community and has to go to an acute setting for an evaluation or emergency stay, then the community-based clinician has a duty to inform the acute placement of the patient's history and needs. And what is and is not appropriate to consider and send back to the community. The responsibility for this transfer of information lies with both sides.

We must also be mindful of how our wise words are interpreted. What clinicians need from, say, an instrumental assessment is not a dietary recommendation but facts on how the swallow mechanism was working, what was impaired, and what approaches helped matters. In an inpatient setting the same clinician is often doing both the assessment and intervention. When patients move between settings different personnel have to work with the data. In some settings, the swallow recommendations are taken as an order – no matter what, Mr Smith should be on thick liquids. This does not inform the team working with the patient and often puts the community-based clinician in a difficult situation – from where we get the familiar feeling of an ethical dilemma.

What's in it for us?

Louis Armstrong once said of jazz that "what we play is life". In dealing with eating and drinking problems we are not technicians measuring absolutes, or even clinicians prescribing the optimal treatment for a disease. Professionals working with people with dysphagia are dealing with a condition that affects life from sustenance to experience and identity (Leslie, 2015). With no other life requirement (air, beating heart, toxin removal, etc.) do we have a say in what, how and with whom we do the thing. This makes dysphagia work one of the most demanding areas in clinical care. It is both biomechanically life threatening, and psychologically the crux of who we see ourselves as and how we relate to our communities. This may be behind our discomfort with refusing or removing feeding tubes which is now firmly established in the legal world as a healthcare intervention like any other which can be refused or withdrawn ("Airedale NHS Trust v Bland," 1993). Nevertheless, speech and language therapists are crucial members of the team working with patients in this field. We cross the boundaries of physical impairment, communicative competence, and experiential context – perhaps we are uniquely qualified to support patients and families in this area. We also have to bear the burden that is the complexity of these decisions for people. Our hope is that you are now willing to step outside of our typical and historical training to view the concepts in this book. Our intent is that by exploring these concepts you will feel better prepared to support your patients and families, more ready to defend your arguments with other professionals and, ideally, sleep a little easier at night.

References

Airedale NHS Trust v Bland, 1 All ER 821 (House of Lords Court of Appeal 1993).

Leslie, P. (2015). Worship the dog not the larynx. Retrieved 23 November 2015, from http://www.dysphagiacafe.com/2015/11/10/worship-the-dog-not-the-larynx/

National Institutes for Health. (2009). Teaching Exploring Bioethics. Retrieved 31 May 2016, from https://science.education.nih.gov/supplements/nih9/bioethics/guide/pdf/Teachers_Guide.pdf

Pretzler, M. (2007). *Pausanias: Travel Writing in Ancient Greece*. London: Duckworth.

Index